Genetic Governance

Health, Risk and Ethics in the Biotech Era

There is currently much interest in the potential transformation of life and new therapeutic opportunities brought about by the so-called genetic revolution. Genetics is increasingly involved in processes of governance that shape the way we see our bodies, ourselves and our environments. Controversy and ethical debate surrounds the use of techniques of cloning, stem cell research and national genetic databases or 'biobanks'. However, there has been little reflection on the socio-political effects of this new genetic knowledge and the changes in practice that are currently impacting on our lives.

Genetic Governance contains contributions from key international researchers who examine the broader issues of genetic debates, look at how prediction and risk assessment is being changed in the arenas of health, medicine and reproduction, and bring new insights on the dangers of surveillance, regulation and increased inequality. This book considers the implications of developments in genetics for contemporary liberal governance, as well as for the future of healthcare and public health.

This book will be invaluable reading for academics and students in health sciences, public health, medical ethics, the sociology of health and illness, science and technology studies, the sociology of the new genetics and political studies.

Robin Bunton is Professor of Sociology at the University of Teesside. He has previously worked as a researcher and practitioner in the public health field and published widely in the sociology of health.

Alan Petersen is Professor of Sociology at the University of Plymouth. He has researched and published widely in the sociology of health and illness, and more specifically in the sociology of the new genetics.

Genetic Governance

Health, Risk and Ethics in the Biotech Era

Edited by

Robin Bunton and Alan Petersen

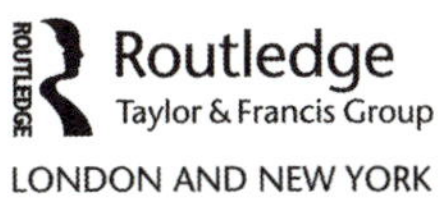
Routledge
Taylor & Francis Group
LONDON AND NEW YORK

First published 2005
by Routledge
2 Park Square, Milton Park, Abingdon, Oxon OX14 4RN

Tel: +44 020 7017 6000
Fax: +44 020 7017 6699

Simultaneously published in the USA and Canada
by Routledge
270 Madison Ave, New York, NY 10016

Routledge is an imprint of the Taylor & Francis Group

Typeset in 10/12 Sabon by Scribe Design Ltd, Ashford, Kent
Printed and bound in Great Britain by TJ International Ltd,
Padstow, Cornwall

British Library Cataloguing in Publication Data
A catalogue record for this book is available from the British Library

Library of Congress Cataloging in Publication Data
A catalog record for this book has been requested

ISBN 0-415-354064 (Hbk)
ISBN 0-415-354072 (Pbk)

Contents

List of contributors

Robin Bunton is Professor of Sociology at the University of Teesside, United Kingdom.

Elizabeth Ettorre is Professor of Sociology and Associate Dean, Faculty of Social Science and Business, University of Plymouth, United Kingdom.

Herbert Gottweis is Professor of Political Science, University of Vienna, Austria.

Ilpo Helén is Academy Research Fellow at the Department of Sociology, University of Helsinki, Finland.

Martha R. Herbert is Assistant Professor of Neurology at Harvard Medical School and Pediatric Neurologist and brain development researcher at the Massachusetts General Hospital, United States.

Piia Jallinoja is a sociologist and senior researcher at the Department of Epidemiology and Health Promotion, National Public Health Institute, Finland.

Susan E. Kelly is Associate Professor of Sociology and Faculty of Epidemiology and Clinical Investigation Sciences at the University of Louisville, United States.

Thomas Lemke is Assistant Professor at Wuppertal University and a Research Fellow at the Institute for Social Research in Frankfurt/Main, Germany.

Alan Petersen is Professor of Sociology at the University of Plymouth, United Kingdom.

Jessica Polzer is a PhD candidate in the Social Science and Health Program, Department of Public Health Sciences, University of Toronto, Canada.

Seppo Poutanen is a researcher in the Department of Sociology at the University of Turku, Finland.

Linda Ward is Director of the Norah Fry Research Centre and Professor of Disability and Social Policy at the University of Bristol, United Kingdom.

Evan Willis is Professor of Sociology and Head of Humanities and Social Sciences on the Albury-Wodonga campus at LaTrobe University in Victoria, Australia.

Acknowledgements

We would like to thank the following people who supported this publication at various stages of its development. Thanks to Barbara Cox and other members of the *Critical Public Health* Editorial Board who supported the idea and initial call for papers. A special thanks to the authors and the referees of the original papers that led to this publication, without whom the project would never have emerged. We would like to thank Taylor & Francis journals publishing team, particularly Janet Remington and Richard Steele, for supporting the idea of the publication and Karen Bowler, Claire Gauler and Cathy Hambly at Routledge for their ongoing assistance. Finally, we extend thanks to Lesley Jones and Ros Porter for their extended support throughout the length of this project.

Genetics and governance

An introduction

Robin Bunton and Alan Petersen

In the early twenty-first century genetics has most definitely entered the popular imagination. Few national newspapers will go longer than a week without reporting on newer 'discoveries', new promises of improvements in health and understanding of our bodies or new ethical dilemmas facing us as a result of developments in genetic research and practice. The announcement, in 2001, that the human genome had been sequenced seems to have marked a decisive point in the development of the genetics so-called revolution. Great expectations await the next wave of research which involves clarification of how genes 'work' (functional genomics), a time that has been dubbed the 'post-genomic' era, which promises to transform concepts of health, illness and the body, and the practices of medicine and public health. New drugs are anticipated which will be 'personalized' to suit our individual gene profiles. Risk analysis will allow greater understanding and management of the contribution of genes to the disease of populations. The enormous promise of the new genetics has also brought substantial concern, critique and comment by lay publics, some scientists, and policy-makers. Innovations such as cloning, the harvesting of embryonic stem cells and genetic databases ('biobanks') have been the subject of considerable controversy and regulatory efforts over recent years. In the wake of Dolly the sheep and other widely publicized genetic research 'breakthroughs', there has been widespread anxiety about the commodification of the body and about the implications of 'tampering with nature', and concern about the adequacy of existing ethical and regulatory safeguards (see e.g. Nelkin and Andrews 1998). While there remains extensive public debate about the rights and wrongs of such developments, there has been less concern for the detailed effects these envisaged changes will have on the ways we make decisions about our bodies and ourselves, our communities and environments; in short on the ways we are governed. This book explores aspects of genetic governance as it pertains to not only the fields of public health and preventive medicine but also broader social existence. It brings together a number of researchers in this international field who attempt to step aside briefly from the ethical problems and dilemmas to explore the current and likely governing effects of the emerging new genetic knowledge and techniques.

As researchers in the social study of health, we were aware of the regulatory and 'governing' features of a number of public health policies, though this potential of public health measures was often unacknowledged by health professionals and policy-makers. Over a number of years we have addressed these issues (Bunton 1992; Bunton et al. 1995, 1997; Petersen and Lupton, 1996; Petersen 1997). We also became aware of the capacity of the new genetics technologies to make incursions into everyday life-worlds and to extend the 'medical gaze' into previously uncharted areas. We have found the work of Michel Foucault a particularly fruitful source of analytic tools and inspiration, in attempting to examine the new forms of surveillance, risk analysis and routine regulation of everyday life (Petersen and Bunton 1997). His work seemed to offer a critical vantage point to address the complex issues emerging from the 'new genetics' in the 1980s and 1990s and yet Foucault's ideas have been relatively unexplored in relation to recent developments in genetics. His work on what he termed 'bio-power' and on the ways that expert knowledge and scientific discourse are drawn upon in the construction of identity seems to offer a way of understanding genetic knowledge and techniques. Foucault's notion of 'governmentality' seems to have particular resonance in the rapidly developing field of genetics and relates to broader questions of rule and the rationale of neoliberal democracies.

Questions of governance in relation to genetics, we contend, include 'ethical, legal, and social' questions. Focusing on governance introduces questions about genetics knowledge and research often left unexplored by recent research on ethical, legal and social issues, and forces us to think more critically about what's at stake in defining a field in this way. With this in mind, we put out a call for submissions to *Critical Public Health* for a special issue on 'Genetic Governance'. The chapters in this volume are revised and updated versions of many of the articles that originally appeared in two issues of *Critical Public Health*, published in 2002 (volume 12, numbers 2 and 3). The contributions address genetic governance, ethics and public health, although we are aware that many of the concerns and issues raised are not restricted to the field of health. These issues have broad social and political implications and are relevant to a wide number of disciplines and fields of study including social care and social policy, crime and criminal justice, international relations, the social study of science and technology and more general sociology. We invited contributions 'addressing issues of social and political regulation, and "genetic-" or "bio-governance" arising from new genetic technologies', particularly those that 'explore and offer critical perspectives on issues of governmentality relating to emerging forms of knowledge and practice'. We made the call in the belief that there is a need for sustained critical and theoretically informed analyses of issues around governance in relation to genetics and public health that had been lacking in the literature. Rapid developments in the field of human genetics pose profound challenges for concepts of governance and ethics. Notions of the natural and the normal have been unsettled substantially. Distinctions such as 'nature' versus 'culture', 'health' versus 'illness', and 'therapy' versus 'enhancement' are questioned by the promises of genetics and a number of genetics-related and other biomedical developments that are already in progress. Recent calls for laws on genetic equality, to outlaw discrimination on the basis of a person's genetic make-up (e.g. Sample 2004), and for 'intergenerational justice', to protect the interests of future generations (e.g. McClean 2004), for example, reveal concerns about the potentially deleterious consequences of such developments and the adequacy of current regulatory frameworks. Through its diverse applications, including agriculture, the military, criminal justice and medicine, genetics is rapidly transforming the nature of political life (Rose 2001). However, we believe that many of the most far-reaching implications of this 'biopolitics' are likely to be seen in the field of public health and preventive medicine.

It was apparent that, although there was a burgeoning literature on the 'ethical, legal and social implications' (ELSI) of new genetic technologies, there appeared to have been little specific theoretical analysis of related issues of governance. Foucault highlighted the close relationship between ethics and governance. He showed the various ways, from Classical Greece to the present, that ethical judgement was implicated in the formation of the self and citizenship. Individuals, he argued, govern themselves through forms of self-care, self-examination and self-discipline, training and exercise. The development of the self and ethical living in relation to sexual morality, for example, depends upon daily practices, routines or techniques for living promoted not only by the Christian Church in Europe but also by modern secular institutions such as the family, the school and the clinic (Foucault 1980). Medical and public health institutions similarly promoted ethics of self-care by promoting a particular 'political anatomy of the body' (Armstrong 1983, 1995).

Foucault's concern with ethical conduct can be contrasted with the philosophical and religious focus on *morality* – a general system of imposed or suggested rules or guides for conduct – and with how the former may provide the basis for breaking with the 'normalizing' tendencies in modern societies. When used in contemporary debates about genetic technologies and other new technologies, however, the term 'ethics' tends to equate with the latter, thus limiting debate about the profound implications of new technologies for how we think about the self and social relations. Thus, the exploration of the 'ethical' implications of the new genetics is often restricted to concerns about confidentiality, informed consent, people's 'right to know or right not to know', who has the right to choose, to 'play God' and so on. Meanwhile, fundamental questions about how people might best relate, and how to nurture 'desirable' forms of self-conduct and social life that are just and equitable receive less attention. In this introduction to the contributions from scholars around the world, we try to sketch out the reason for a focus on governance before examining the particular contribution Michel Foucault's work makes to this task, particularly his work on governmentality and the links he made between issues of ethics and governance. We argue for an integration of ethics and governance before discussing the recent interest in governance and its relevance to the study of genetics. We introduce the various contributions within this focus referring to the more micro processes of the construction of the self and then the strategies for governing populations and identities. Finally, we reflect on the nature of genetic knowledge and some likely areas for future research.

Governance

The varied contributions to this volume illustrate the diverse meanings of the notion of governance. Treatments of governance can be found in a wide range of disciplines including sociology, social and public policy analysis, international relations, economics, systems analysis and political science. Like many fields of scholarship, the use of key concepts is influenced by disciplinary backgrounds, particular theoretical and empirical concerns and many other contextual and political influences that constitute domain assumptions. Though interest in this area has grown considerably since the early 1980s, the etymology of the word 'governance' can be traced to the Greek verb *Kubernan*, meaning to pilot or steer, and which led to the Latin *gubernare*, also connoting piloting, rule-making or steering (Kjaer 2004). This term was to be associated with the arts of nation-state government but more latterly has come to be viewed more broadly as systems of rule at all levels of human activity, from family relations to international organization (Rosenau 1995). Crucially, the term refers to the stewardship of 'the rules of the game' and guiding or organizing a number of actors, from a distance. Contemporary interest in governance reflects recognition that the contemporary world is influenced and structured by something more than state rule. Contemporary analysis of governance focuses on the roles of networks of organizations, institutions and actors in pursuit of common and competing goals, working at local, national and transnational levels and transgressing any state–society divide. Public sector reform was endemic in Western countries in the latter part of the twentieth century, with agendas of privatization, decentralization and shifts in the principles of public involvement and participation. National government functions were transferred to lower regional levels on the one hand and to supranational organizations on the other, creating a more pluralistic and often fragmented public sector. Governance seemed to offer a perspective on the emerging forms of organization of the patterns of services. In the health care systems of these

Western countries there has a been a notable tendency to redistribute responsibility from state health care systems not only towards private service providers but also to individuals, who are increasingly expected and encouraged to manage their own health by careful choices and actively reducing lifestyle risks. Ironically this individualizing of health has been led by 'public' health care regimes that have sought to activate responsible citizenship and 'empower' communities and draw them into a network of actors working alongside local and international commerce to maximize health.

Recently, then, governance has been used to make sense of rapid global, socio-cultural developments that appear to have decentred notions of the supremacy of the nation-state in determining forms of health and welfare regulation since the late 1970s. The state's ability to underwrite social citizenship by social programmes designed to ameliorate the harsher effects of the needs of capital has been threatened (Williams 2002; Ginsberg 1998), it has been argued, and we live in an increasingly risky, 'runaway world' (Giddens 1991) threatened by unpredictable global forces and processes. Established features of state-led health and welfare have been reviewed and restructured and a number of cherished principles, such as the pursuit of universal needs and sustained economic growth and full employment, have been questioned at the onset of what has become known as neoliberalism.

In these new economic and social circumstances health governance must be considered in broad terms which encompass the entire social system, the conduct of individual life, and the interrelationships between collective and self governance. Statements and analyses of international developments in health policy and public health illustrate an emerging interest in health governance alongside health reform (World Health Organization (WHO) 1998; Lavis and Sullivan 1999). 'Good' governance for health has placed emphasis upon health development and systems-based interventions (particularly integrated and effective healthy public policies), held to be more efficient in producing population health gain, especially among more disadvantaged and vulnerable groups, than individually orientated programmes. There is a belief that health contributes to social and economic development and that development likewise enhances good health. The UK Labour Party's Third-Way doctrine emphasizes the 'joined-up', cross-sector collaborative strength in health and social care strategy in such a way that the needs of capital and social need are aligned.

Much of such focus on health governance is stronger on vision than critique. It tends to attribute significant potential for control and democratic process in a new world order, which involves new forms of governance, despite some evidence to the contrary. In February 2004 the United Kingdom Chancellor of the Exchequer Gordon Brown warned that the developed world was failing on its promise to reduce global poverty and sickness. Brown was reflecting a concern from the World Economic Forum that the United Nations (UN) Millennium Development Goals are faltering and failing to provide 'globalization for all'. The activities of cross-national instruments such as The General Agreement on Trade in Services (GATS) and the World Trade Organization (WTO) have been able to reduce local and national concerns for social products such as health to mere 'externalities' in ways that undermine global health governance strategies and threaten health. Moreover, Trade Related Intellectual Property Rights (TRIPS) agreements can benefit corporate interests to the detriment of local health governance strategies. Such agreements are particularly important in relation to the development of the newer genetic technologies. Intellectual property laws, for example, can act as a way of transforming indigenous knowledge and genetic resources into profitable commodities (Whitt 1998: 35). Exploitation by 'knowledge-rich economies' of the traditional bio-knowledge stock is potentially very profitable, promising the development of newer drugs and health-related commodities. Exploitation of such stocks by Western corporations, however, is likely to exacerbate disparities in wealth and health between the countries of the North and the South. Indigenous groups have objected to such 'bio-prospecting' and opposed 'bio-colonialism' that the new genetic technologies and intellectual property right laws have made possible (Petersen and Bunton 2002). Despite regular failures of global health governance, however, its potential as a new 'political space' in which to build public health continues to be championed (Kickbusch 2004).

Some of the problems associated with health governance illustrate broader problems with the notions of governance itself, at least as the term has been taken up in certain aspects of the study of public policy, comparative policy analysis and international relations. There is a noticeable positive or perhaps even idealistic bias to the study of governance. While stressing the pursuit of common values and a state–society synergy it can too often focus on 'winners' rather than 'losers' in the networking processes (Kjaer 2004). Networks typically have limited representativeness and 'exclusions' from the processes of governance tend to be underplayed, as do the conflicts with the processes of governance. Hirst (2000) has noted that while democratic institutions are designed to manage conflict, networks of governance are not. There is a danger in underplaying the ways in which powerful interests can manipulate and interrupt processes of participation in governance. In the final chapter, Herbert Gottweis illustrates nicely how to avoid such one-sided analysis describing the rise of industry as a powerful force in the genomics governance network.

Governmentality and ethics

Theoretical perspectives on issues of governance included here are diverse. Our own interest in the work of Foucault was shared by some of the contributors. Foucault's contribution to the study of health and the body has been profound and his work on the link between scientific discourse and governance has opened up the way for an enormous number of lines of inquiry. Foucault saw the government of biological needs as a central feature of modernity. In a number of studies he described the control and modification of life processes – birth, death, sexual and blood relations, health and disease, etc. – as forms of government that supplanted that of sovereign rule. From the eighteenth century onwards the 'life sciences' became implicated in the governance of populations and individuals. In his *History of Sexuality* (Volume One), he described the emergence of 'bio-power' in the eighteenth century as 'without doubt an indispensable element in the development of capitalism' (Foucault 1980: 140–141). Sciences such as biology became central to the apparatus of political rule, as it was increasingly subject to scientific calculation in order to make bodies more disciplined and useful for the emergent capitalist order. There was an increasing preoccupation with matters of health, modes of subsistence and living conditions, and with the regulation of sexuality as the notion of public health was being born (Rosen 1993[1958]).

This was also the period of the 'birth of the clinic' (Foucault 1975). As Foucault notes, eugenics, too, was integral to the effort to transform life. The concern with 'purity of the blood' implied an extension and intensification of power over bodies, and the claim to have a 'superior blood' 'implied both the systematic genocide of others and the risk of exposing oneself to a total sacrifice' (Foucault 1980: 150). The drive to measure, categorize and hierarchize biological phenomena were aspects of what Foucault referred to as a 'normalizing society', which was 'the historical outcome of a technology of power centred on life' (Foucault 1980: 144). The life sciences became part of a new mechanism of power that:

> Permits time and labour, rather than wealth and commodities, to be extracted from bodies. It is a type of power which is constantly exercised by means of surveillance rather than in a discontinuous manner by means of a system of levies and obligations distributed over time. It presupposes a tightly knit grid of material coercions rather than the physical existence of a sovereign.
>
> (Foucault 1980: 14)

These material coercions consisted of disciplines aimed at the individual body on the one hand, and the population on the other. Foucault developed a relational view of power that throws into question some of the assumptions of a singular, top-down domination involving state institutions and ruling groups or classes. Instead his work forces us to consider the practices, networks and techniques that constitute contemporary modes of power and regulation.

Rose (2001) takes up Foucault's insistence that we live in a 'biopolitical' age and that new configurations of power have taken place in Western societies that rely on the governance of 'life itself'. For Rose this involves political strategies that attempt to track and regulate risk. He sees two main state-sponsored biopolitical strategies that were apparent in the twentieth century. The first is the hygienist programmes, which were typical of a strategy to instil habits and moral health to maximize the fitness of the general population, but particularly the poor. The second sought to maximize the fitness of the population, but through privileging one site – that of reproduction. This strategy included eugenics that sought to improve the body politic and relieve it of the economic and social burdens of disease and degeneracy. By contrast Rose notes that contemporary biopolitics differs however, in that it is no longer tied to the ideals of the state, which takes charge of individual lives in 'the name of the destiny of all' (Rose 2001: 3–5). Today's biopolitical strategies are far more diverse and encompass many national cultures, many identities and many communities, in line with the more diverse political regimes of neoliberalism. The governance of 'life-itself' takes place in multiple sites with multiple mechanisms of rule that involve the actions and relations between entrepreneurs, clinicians, researchers, active citizens and communities, professions, governments and a great many more actors. Some documentation of this variety in the networks of genetic governance can be found in the accounts of the development of genomics in a number of countries. Fujimura (2003) describes how Japanese genomics has been developed with a particular vision or 'imagined' set of social relations or 'globally defined possibilities' that reinvent East–West relationships. Such analysis illustrates how genetic scientists are socio-cultural entrepreneurs with particular agendas in building what Latour (1987) has referred to as socio-technical networks.

Foucault's work has been taken up by recent scholars to describe the rationale and the practice of neoliberalism with a particular focus on political processes 'beyond the state' and the notion of governmentality (Dean 1999; Rose 1999). The concept of governmentality was developed by Foucault in the latter part of his life, and focuses attention on rationalities and practices or the 'arts' of governance. As Gordon notes:

> A rationality of government will thus mean a way or system of thinking about the nature of the practice of government (who can govern; what governing is; what or who is governed), capable of making some form of that activity thinkable and practicable both to its practitioners and to those upon whom it was practiced.
>
> (Gordon 1991: 3)

It involves the idea of the nature of 'conduct' in all its locations. In Chapter 4 Jessica Polzer draws directly on this notion in addressing genetic testing and citizenship responsibility. A governmentality perspective helps us to see the knowledge and practices of the new genetics in public health in sites as varied as state policy-making, the commercial activities of the biotech industry, the shaping of biomedical research, the creation of genetic norms and ideas of genetic risk, clinical practice (in genetic testing clinics for example), the education and training of specialist genetic professionals, and in the practices of self-governance by which individuals seek out and use genetic risk information to regulate their own behaviour (such as reproductive choices). Like Rose, Polzer argues that whereas the practices of the 'old eugenics' relied upon state-directed coercive regulatory strategies targeting those deemed 'genetically unfit', contemporary forms of genetic testing are typical of neoliberal governmentality that rely on more opaque practices of self-monitoring and self-regulation.

In presenting the work of this group of scholars, we found it useful to divide it into two aspects of governance of genomics. In discussing 'bio-power' Foucault (1980) made a distinction between the regulatory effects of power/knowledge that centred on the individual body and sought to optimize its capacities, exerting force and maximizing its usefulness, and included self-disciplinary measures and behavioural regulation, and the regulation of the population. Technologies at this latter level seek to regulate both moralities and maximize health potential and longevity by controlling groups of people. These two realms of power over life are not mutually exclusive. Clearly individual regulation of health risk by single acts of restricted reproduction following genetic testing, for example, have a population effect and attempts at population-wide regulation require individual acts of regulation and discipline. We have grouped the chapters in this volume into three parts according to their primary focus. Part I 'Ethics, risk and governance', consists of chapters that begin their analysis from the 'anatomo politics' of the individual body and the techniques that forge identity formation and active citizenship and governance. Part II, 'Risk, population and identity', deals with issues of inequalities that are being perpetuated by the construction and privileging of different social groupings. Part III, 'Knowledge, governance and the future', includes three chapters that reflect on some ideological and epistemological issues and also some reflection on the future of genetic governance.

Ethics, risk and governance

Chapter 1 illustrates the intimate relationship between ethical considerations and governance. Piia Jallinoja examines the arguments and practices of medical ethics as part of a network of experts, codes, regulations and morals. Ethics are described as a set of practices tied up in the processes of medicine, legislation and the health care system rather than as simply an abstract entity. There is no single site for ethics in medicine; rather it appears as verbalized or written codes, arguments or practices, and made concrete in medical technologies such as screening projects and physician–patient interactions in genetic counselling. This chapter examines three decades during which medical ethics gradually became a part of Finnish genetic testing, screening and counselling by looking at one institution founded in 1971 and three genetic counselling and screening programmes in the 1990s. The year 1970 was an important one as it was the year that liberal abortion law came into force and during the following years the organization of medical genetics services was activated. In 1971 the position of physician specialist in medical genetics was founded at the Family Federation of Finland, and in 1972 the first professorship in medical genetics in Finland was founded at the University of Helsinki. The chapter does not seek to offer a better ethical standpoint but to stand back and examine the forms and content of medical ethics: how ethics and the correctness of genetic screening were discussed and argued, and how and by whom the ethics was verified and especially how ethics was integrated into local medical research and practice. As Jallinoja argues, medico-ethical practices are unable to solve the moral dilemmas of selective abortion, and other issues concerning life, that make choice about tests and abortion so difficult for many people.

Jallinoja's chapter nicely illustrates the local acts of governance that begin to follow from the establishment of new systems and networks of medical knowledge, practice and technology. It provides a detailed account of the establishment of socio-technical systems that draw upon the newer genetic knowledge and techniques. Here we are shown the processes by which medical ethics became 'operationalized' and integrated in the processes of screening and decisions surrounding pregnancy and termination. Medical staff have a need to evaluate public acceptance of 'voluntary decisions' and 'freedoms' and whether freedom of choice has been exercised. This is by no means a simple issue.

In Chapter 2 Ilpo Helén also addresses issues of ethics and choice in relation to advanced techniques of antenatal screening (including genetic testing) in maternity care in Finland. Like Jallinoja, Helén is aware of the complexity of issues surrounding the 'imperative' of risk rationality that newer knowledge brings with it. This is a problem for the sharing of knowledge and individual choice not only in perinatal decisions but also in broader issues of knowledge, trust and scientific 'reflexivity' related to the 'risk society'. Beck's account of scientific reflexivity offers an optimistic account of the effects of reflexive awareness of risk, which is questioned to some degree by both Helén and Jallinoja. They point to the problematic issues of 'freedom' and 'choice' in these circumstances exemplified by a number of authors (Rose 1999) who point out that states of freedom and autonomy are not free from power. 'Selective abortion', Helén argues, exemplifies the ways in which problems involved in the implementation of high-tech biomedicine in clinical practice and primary health care are defined as *ethical*. Furthermore, selective abortion and the related ethical controversies are embedded in emerging forms of bio-power, or *vital politics* (Lemke 2000; Rose 2001). While the emergence of new forms of governance of 'life-itself' is engendered by newer discourses and new socio-technical regimes, the tendency is to present these in terms of risk and to emphasize health and life as matters of individuality and selfhood.

Helén's chapter examines different settings in which questions of foetal diagnosis are defined as ethical ones, arguing that the ethical problem varies from one context of 'ethicalization' to another. The study is based on an analysis of the discourse on the implementation of high-tech foetal diagnosis and antenatal screening in Finnish maternity care drawing upon analysis of articles and other writings by Finnish physicians in Finnish and international medical journals on the subjects of antenatal screenings and diagnosis, as well as reviews by Finnish medical geneticists on developments in and prospects for their field.

The choices and anxieties that pregnant women face in the procedures of antenatal diagnosis and selective abortion exemplify the ethical problems involved in medical technology and advanced biomedicine. Widespread adoption of informed consent and non-directiveness as the guiding principles of foetal diagnosis, genetic research and counselling, stem cell research and of collecting samples and medical information for biobanks is an indication of the need to make state-of-the-art medical technology ethically acceptable. Articulation of problems and controversies in terms of ethics overshadows political aspects of the development of genetic technologies. This case study illustrates high-tech health care's capacity for prediction and promise that conceives of diagnosis of 'potential disease' and the risks of 'ill-health', irrespective of any symptoms. It defines the 'molecular destiny of the person' and offers options to overcome and change the destiny of an individual based upon prediction and promise, and demands a person live his or her own life beforehand, extending our capacity for 'care of the self' (Foucault 1990). Helén relates this advanced form of *responsibilization*, made possible by the new technology, to broader issues of risk and choice discussed by others (Beck-Gernsheim 1995: 289–290; O'Malley 1996; Petersen 1999; Novas and Rose 2000: 502–507).

As issues of choice and freedom are becoming more important in the governance of genetics, so processes of public consultation, decision-making and accountability are achieving growing significance. In Chapter 3, Seppo Poutanen draws upon a study of the launch of genetic screening in Finland, which he views as an emerging form of liberal governance. He considers the potential of Bayesian decision analysis to aid decision-making in the context of uncertainty generated by risk information. Although, according to Poutanen, the view that Bayesian decision analysis can form part of the solution is speculative, he suggests that it may be promoted as a useful tool in bioethical practice.

According to proponents of the so-called new genetics, genetic information will greatly facilitate the diagnosis and prediction of diseases, and thereby improve treatment or enhance prevention of illness. Consequently, both lay populations and health care and public health workers are being called upon to become 'genetically literate' (Petersen and Bunton 2002: 6, 28, 33, 52, 56–57). At the level of the individual, an anticipated burgeoning number of genetic tests is expected to assist in the identification of 'susceptible' individuals or those destined to develop disease (e.g. Huntington's disease, cystic fibrosis), while at the population level, research involving large-scale genetic databases is anticipated to generate information that will allow the identification of genetically 'at risk' groups within the population. The former presumed benefits are in medicine – which proponents argue will become more 'predictive' and 'personalized' – while the latter are in public health. (The distinction between these fields is becoming blurred with the 'geneticization' of health.) According to proponents of genetic technologies in health care and public health, the provision of predictive or risk information will enhance the autonomy of the individual. Individuals, it is argued, may undertake necessary lifestyle changes to reduce the probability of developing disease or plan their lives with greater certainty about their futures. The premise that more information provides more choice and thus enhances autonomy is widely held as an unproblematic given by many professionals within public health and medicine. However, it bears close examination.

To begin, there are a range of questions pertaining to the rationalities of government and practices of the self associated with the provision of personal genetic information, especially through genetic counselling. Technologies such as genetic tests and genetic databases, and genetic knowledge, constitute identities and create new ways of seeing and acting upon bodies and selves. People who are diagnosed with a mutant gene become classified as the 'pre-symptomatically ill' who should manage their relationship to risks. Genetic diagnosis creates categories of the genetically 'at risk' or diseased and the reproductively unfit who are subjects of medical, legal and state intervention and who are called upon to plan their present in light of expectations about what their genetic endowment may hold (Novas and Rose 2000: 487–488). What forms of sociality – or 'biosociality' (Rabinow 1992) – have emerged or are emerging as a consequence of the 'geneticization' of health? Technologies generate their own imperatives, in terms of surveillance and 'treatment' or risk management, and imply certain forms of action and relationship with self and others. Ultrasound and other technologies used in prenatal care, including genetic technologies, offer new ways of perceiving and surveilling foetuses (Hartouni 1997). Decisions about termination and about diet, for example, are shaped by the use of technologies of prenatal screening. As genetic technologies become routinized in health care and public health, it becomes difficult for publics to resist their use and implied actions when they are widely seen to be beneficial. With a focus on 'health' as a valued ideal in many contemporary societies, and growing consumerism in health care more generally (see Henderson and Petersen 2002), there is an expectation that 'responsible' citizens will want to play their part in using whatever supposedly beneficial technologies are available. Practitioners are also under great compulsion to use genetic technologies because of pressures from parents to have a 'perfect' baby, and also because of fears about litigation, for example for 'wrongful birth' (Malinowski 1994). Thus, they become 'willing' participants in the technology of genetic surveillance. They not only partake in the governance of their 'patients', but also constitute and govern themselves as 'responsible', 'law-abiding' practitioners. In short, genetic technologies and knowledge can be seen to shape the ways of thinking and acting of all parties involved. In this context, the notion of autonomy within ethics seems rather limited and limiting, and denies the power relations at work in defining a condition as 'genetic-related' and as in need of technological intervention.

Ethical debates, such as 'the right to know versus the right not to know' about one's genetic risk status (e.g. Chadwick et al. 1997) and 'rights and responsibilities in the face of genetic knowledge' (e.g. Rhodes 2002), reveal and convey a view of human subjects as unconstrained rational decision-makers, thereby denying the profound influence of socio-cultural and political contexts on thinking and conduct. They deny the discursive link between 'risk' and responsibility and the assumption that responsible citizens will keep themselves informed about genes, inheritance and health (Petersen 1999: 122–123). There is a need for analyses of how ethics knowledge constructs human subjects, their capabilities and their limitations, and how the prescriptions and practices of ethics (e.g. ethics codes and committees) shape fields of action in public health and preventive medicine. Foucault would likely have drawn attention to practices of power and truth games underpinning bioethics and questioned bioethicists' claims to be necessarily 'helping' people (see Frank and Jones 2003: 184–185). His work leads to such questions as: how does the identification of a disease as inherited and inheritable shape subjectivity (i.e. 'awareness of self')? What forms of (self-)surveillance are implied by practices of managing genetic risk? What scope is there for subjects to negotiate or contest the imperatives surrounding the use of genetic technologies and the provision of genetic information in medical and public health settings? Foucault would reject the bioethics concept of the 'autonomous self' who 'chooses' to place him- or herself within a hierarchical therapeutic relationship for his or her own good, as required by medical power relations (Frank and Jones 2003: 185), and instead interrogate the very language of bioethics, including concepts such as 'choice', 'autonomy', 'rights', 'beneficence', 'altruism', 'justice' and so on, for what it reveals about concepts of self and society and implied relations of power. There is a need to examine how the language of genetic citizenship (Petersen and Bunton 2002: Chapter 7; Petersen 2003a) shapes how subjects define themselves and conduct their relationships (see also Rose and Novas 2004), and serves to orient action along some avenues to the neglect of others, for example environmental reforms. The value and limitations of the concept and language of human rights, developed within Western liberal democracies, in particular need investigation. Debates about the human rights and social justice implications of developments in biotechnology and genetic research often draw upon universalist and 'essentialist' conceptions of human nature and of the individual (see e.g. Burley 1999; Fukuyama 2003: Chapters 7, 8; Habermas 2003) that are questioned by the very developments that are described.

In Chapter 4 Jessica Polzer adopts a Foucauldian approach to examine a number of features of the 'geneticization' of aspects of social life focusing on the discourses of 'genetic risk'. Risk is linked to governance here as it has appeared in a number of post-Foucauldian studies. Castel's often-quoted work refers to the ways in which contemporary professionals are concerned less with the treatment of 'dangerous individuals' than with the flow of a range of populations at risk (Castel 1991). In describing 'biopolitics', Rose (2001) notes the centrality of risk-thinking, or 'risk-politics', which consists of ways of identifying levels of risk across populations and also of identifying 'high-risk' groups in need of risk management. This type of analysis has featured in work applied to public health to highlight its regulatory potential (Bunton et al. 1995; Petersen and Lupton 1996; Gastaldo 1997; Nettleton 1997). There are interesting similarities to be found in the roots of both governance and risk. They share an ancient Greek origin and a nautical connotation. The understanding of risk has shifted from earlier general notions of risk as probability relating to the play of natural forces to that pertaining today which tends to have connotations of danger and the potential for harm associated with human action (Wildavsky 1988). Though emerging in mathematical calculations regarding gambling and used in the seventeenth century to try to insure maritime ventures, the idea of risk appears to have been derived from its roots from the Greek word '*rhiza*', which also referred to the hazards of sailing the seas, the dangers of cliffs, winds and tides and the potential for avoiding such harm. Both terms imply some 'reasoned' commitment to the control over human society and over nature. This concern can be seen in the recent interest in risk and health within social science.

The Janus-faced nature of risk has been noted, and its ability to make population-based calculations accountable in individual terms, as individuals assume responsibility for a range of health risks such as coronary heart disease, by limiting their fat intake and taking exercise (or at least feeling guilty when they do not) (Lupton 1999). Polzer documents processes by which active citizenship is accomplished, as individuals participate in informed decision-making during genetic testing. Individuals are expected to exercise their rights to demand access to genetic testing services and learn about their 'genetic risk', and subsequently modify their lifestyles. In doing so they become willing self-governing citizens, perform their 'freedom' in ways that casts them as responsible citizens who actively take charge of their health through personal and familial risk management. The processes of predictive genetic testing construct citizens as 'carriers' of health risk and constitute the family as the 'natural link' between the personal ethic of maintaining good health and more general political objectives. This establishes risk within a web of 'genetic connectedness' (Novas and Rose 2000) which demarcates 'the family' as a territory of government.

Risk, population and identity

Some of the macro concerns with genetic governance, or what Foucault referred to as the 'biopolitics of population', reflect fears about the resurgence of eugenics in the late twentieth century. In recent years, there has been a growing body of social research on the implications of genetics and genomics. In the United Kingdom, the ESRC (Economic and Social Research Council) Genomics Network, launched in 2002, has spawned a range of new genetics/genomics research projects and scholarly exchanges. Work thus far has been diverse and has often been largely descriptive. Much of this research is inattentive to questions of history and politics, especially global political-economy, and to the historical and cultural specificity of concepts and terms which are often used as though their meanings are widely shared or even self-evident, when in fact they are not. For example, the term 'new genetics' is often used as though there is general agreement on its meaning, denying its lack of definitional clarity (Petersen and Bunton 2002: 36–39). Similarly, 'bioethics' is often taken as designating a field of established knowledge, when in fact the question of what constitutes this field (which, in the event, has a history of little more than three decades) is one of considerable ongoing debate and contestation (see e.g. Engelhardt 2000: 1–4; Haimes 2002). We believe that recent developments in genetics call for novel theoretical approaches and research questions, and a more critical approach to language and discourse. In particular, they call for greater attention to the politics of knowledge about genetics and to examination of the power relations at work in claims made about the value and implications of genetic research. The uncritical use of the term 'the *new* genetics' evident in much recent social science literature, for instance, suggests a decisive break with the past and denies how 'new' may serve as a boundary marker and bolster professional power, by demarcating the field, which is assumed to be progressive and 'empowering', and differentiating it from that that is assumed to be pseudo-scientific and coercive, i.e. 'old' eugenics. This denies the diversities of the forms of eugenics in their histories and the continuities between 'new genetic' and 'eugenic' practices (Petersen and Bunton 2002: 39–45). Similarly, the unproblematic use of 'bioethics' to signify a field of scholarship and practice, which suggests consensus on the field's content and boundaries, can divert attention from the historical and cultural specificity of 'ethics' in relation to biomedicine and the interests at stake (see Jallinoja, Chapter 1). Although often portrayed as being politically neutral, 'bioethical' knowledge and practice reveals a particular conception of the human subject and of science and society, and can constitute part of the technology of governance in that it may serve to delimit fields of action and to fulfil certain governmental objectives.

In the opening chapter of Part II (Chapter 5) Thomas Lemke also draws directly upon Foucault's notion of governmentality, examining the shift from eugenics to the government of genetic risks. He shows how genetic knowledge and genetic technologies are used in the government of individuals and populations, how medical practices and diagnostic tools function as political technologies on the one hand and as moral technologies on the other. He uses this to address the distinction made between the eugenics movements of the early twentieth century and those of the new genetics at the turn of the twenty-first. Lemke examines parallels and differences in genetic practices today and those that typified the excesses of the 'old genetics'. He places at the heart of these debates the fear that there will be a re-emergence, return or a 'backdoor to eugenics' (Duster 2003). Lemke takes us a little deeper into the argument here, noting that it is no longer sufficient to criticize the 'biologization of society', as the dichotomy between nature and culture is getting more problematic, a theme taken up since the early 1990s in much social science (Haraway 1991; Latour 1993; Williams et al. 2003). Following Rheinberger (2000), Lemke argues that the natural and the social can no longer be seen as ontologically different and that it is not tenable to assume a rupture between the 'old' and the 'new' genetics. The techniques of the new genetics, such as genetic testing and reproductive counselling, might comprise practices that extend beyond the 'racial hygiene' strategies of eugenics in the name of the optimization of human capital, self-determination and individual freedom. Rather than building a 'new' (or even post-) genetics, we might well be entering an era of the 'eugenics of risk', it is argued, which make the old distinctions irrelevant.

A number of social studies in the late 1990s developed critiques of genetics that focused upon the tendency of genetics to reduce complex causes of health conditions to oversimplistic genetic origins (in the search for the 'gene' responsible for alcohol addiction or homosexuality), the individualizing of a number of socially constructed phenomena (such as intelligence) and the 'essentializing' of variations in human capacities (Marteau and Richards 1996). Behind such concerns is the fear of increased discrimination against groups of people such as disabled populations or those 'at risk' of developing certain health conditions. Genetic knowledge can reproduce inequality by identifying populations and by informing processes of exclusion, coercion or elimination. A number of chapters in this volume illustrate this concern. Inequality engendered by the new genetic knowledge and techniques are a particular focus of the chapters by Ettorre, Ward and Kelly. The strategies for this regulation are various and involve aspects of risk management, exclusion, and the fabrication of identities.

The themes of risk and surveillance are taken up by Elizabeth Ettorre in Chapter 6, which conceptualizes the links between reproduction, gender and bodies in relation to the introduction of the new genetics. This chapter draws upon data from the complex socio-technical system involved in the organization and use of genetic tests for prenatal diagnosis, drawing upon an empirical study of European experts. Ettorre addresses the mobilization of genetics through the idea of surveillance medicine and describes how a mechanistic view of the human body is privileged in techniques of reproductive genetics. While echoing many of the issues of governance found in Polzer's treatment of risk, her critical perspective is drawn largely from sociology of health and illness and from feminist critiques of reproductive medicine and highlights the propensity of the new genetics to focus on women's physical bodies in order to reproduce 'good' genetic capital which represents a further 'medicalization' of the reproductive process. Reproductive genetics appears to exert more restraint and impose more limitations on women's than men's bodies. Ettorre calls for more sociological engagement to counter the over-privileging of genetic knowledge in reproduction. Such engagement will problematize the use of routine notions of risk and risk reduction.

The social study of surveillance medicine has stressed the regulatory potential of the medical gaze. Enhanced by genetic technologies, this gaze can facilitate strategies of identification and manipulation of different subpopulations, as well as processes of exclusion. In Chapter 7, Linda Ward takes up issues of identity ascription and exclusion relating to the new genetics and people with learning difficulties asking, whose right to choose? Arguably one of the groups most affected by developments such as prenatal testing and counselling, people with learning disabilities have largely been absent from this public discourse, and thus excluded from full citizenship rights. Routinization of prenatal testing is frequently assumed to be integral to improvements in prenatal care, despite the anticipated outcome being the selective abortion of foetuses detected as having impairment. The chapter explores some of the fundamental issues, assumptions and contradictions hidden in 'normal practice' in this area, and the tension between two apparent goals of prenatal testing programmes: the extension of parental choice and a commitment to impairment prevention.

In her chapter, Ward reviews some critical arguments put forward by disabled people on the implications of the new genetics and developments in prenatal testing for disability rights. Disability activists and scholars have long challenged the potential of genetic knowledge and technology to medicalize disability, particularly when framed in terms of prenatal 'choice' (Bailey 1996). Such concerns are reminiscent of the cruder exclusions of the era of eugenics rather than contemporary forms of governance (though these two forms of governance may not be mutually exclusive). The nature of 'choice' becomes critical, as do the technological and ideological influences over such 'choice'. Shakespeare (1998) has referred to the emphasis on non-coercive choice in prenatal genetic counselling as a type of 'weak eugenics'. The notion of choice may have insidious consequences once it enters popular culture. More recently, he has noted the potential for disability, once genetic testing is generally accepted, to become associated with 'irresponsible parental choice' (Shakespeare 2003). An alternative future is also quite possible. The increased awareness that we all carry 'defective' genes could produce a climate in which we accept that 'we are all disabled now'. Shakespeare and Ward's arguments here highlight the potential of genetic techniques to make certain views of the world appear 'natural' or beyond question. Technologies have the capacity to solidify and make such contingent patterns of social relationship appear solid, even intentional. Like ideologies, they can frame a particular view of health, disease, life and nature, justifying new sets of relationship and new forms of governance (Petersen and Bunton 2002). This point is made very clear in the treatment of social class.

In Chapter 8, Susan E. Kelly analyses the ways in which the 'naturalization' of class inequality may be accomplished by geneticized debates about the idea of a 'genetic underclass' in the United States. She explores the usefulness of this metaphor for framing genetics and social disadvantage. The notion of a genetic underclass has been conceptualized as an 'economically segregated, biologically inferior, socially and politically marginalized status emerging from inequities of access to genetic health benefits or genetic enhancements'. Drawing upon analysis of in-depth interviews with mothers of children affected with a genetic condition or illness, she considers the notion of a genetic underclass as it has appeared in medical ethics and policy literatures and argues that little direct evidence to support the idea of a genetically unemployable or uninsurable underclass, though theoretical dimensions associated with the underclass do suggest ways of examining dynamics of genetic conditions and social disadvantage. Kelly identifies issues and processes of importance to understanding relationships between social disadvantage and public health genetics. Her chapter explores the ways or mechanisms through which social inequalities can be reproduced through the application of reproductive genetic technologies, which may contribute to the emergence of a 'genetic underclass'. She argues for policy to prevent the geneticization of inequality in relation to families with children with genetic disabilities.

Knowledge, governance and the future

Part III of this book considers the development of genetic knowledge and research, as well as potential future scenarios. The production of knowledge, disciplinary structures and technologies lies at the heart of governance in late modern 'knowledge-rich' economies. Our three concluding chapters examine the production of knowledge in a number of ways.

Evan Willis in Chapter 9 examines the effects of the new genetic knowledge on one field of endeavour – that of public health. To address this very broad field he takes three case studies – ozone and the melanoma gene, bladder cancer and chemical workers, and haemochromatosis – and observes the different complexions on the framing and intervention that genetic knowledge brings to these topics. In doing so he points to the dangers of the geneticization of public health as a field of academic study. He points also to complexity of this field of knowledge and practice and how concepts of environment, individual and agent can be affected by the introduction of genetic techniques, thereby raising issues of the weighting of environment over individual and collective choice in public matters and indicates how social context influences the ways in which these traditional tensions in public health are resolved. Willis asks, 'If advances in the understanding of the genetic basis of disease have outpaced the related understanding of the social and societal implications, how can social scientists contribute to the evolution of policies to guide and regulate the new genetically based technologies, their development, practices and the uses to which they are put?' Public health, like other fields, must encounter the growth in genetic knowledge and make assessments of its uses. At the turn of the twentieth century advances in microbiology and of the emerging eugenics movement were to have a profound effect on public health (Petersen and Bunton 2002). It would seem that a repeat encounter is afoot a century later with a return of sociobiological explanations of health and disease.

In Chapter 10, Martha Herbert reflects upon developments in genetic research itself and argues that in-depth understanding undermines the notion that genes are the key to organismic development and pathology. While DNA dogma continues to inform public opinion and corporate investment strategies often determine research, the shortfalls in the science are salutary and current developments in the field suggest new frameworks for research and for understanding the organism. The dominance of 'gene thinking' in biology, she argues, has had an intellectual and economic imperative that seeks commodification and supports a reductionist model of biological reality. Herbert suggests that this period of dominance is coming to an end and that questioning of geneticization is needed to understand the success of the gene model. Her conclusions here match those of theorists examining governance and knowledge in advanced liberal societies. By making choices about the nature of the knowledge we promote and develop, we are ultimately influencing the type of governance we accomplish with effects upon social relationships, self-understanding and self-construction and ultimately, as Rose (2001) reminds us, life itself.

Finally Chapter 11, by Herbert Gottweis, returns to the theme of governance and illustrates how an analysis of the governance of genomics (or even post-genomics) can highlight the conflicts and workings of power and interest inherent in particular socio-technical networks. Gottweis notes an initial lack of conflict within the field of genomics policy. He acknowledges that current political arenas are populated by many relatively autonomous actors creating patterns of structured co-operation despite the absence of a central organizing authority and describes the emerging structure of governance in the field of genomics and the different ways genomic research has been supported and regulated by governmental agencies in a number of Western and non-Western countries. In his account we see the rise of the genomics industry as a powerful force in the genomics governance network and the challenges that face this much admired, though highly controversial sector which is introducing a number of fundamental transformations in the practices of modern biology and medicine, in society and culture. He observes that the essence of governance is to reach social compromise and binding decisions, which should involve policy-makers, scientists and entrepreneurs, patients, consumers, the general public, the media and others. The government is but one actor among many in shaping biomedical futures.

While the transformations brought about by genomics have created a number of policy challenges, Gottweis notes that there exists a 'cultural vacuum' which gives rise to generalized public anxiety about the implications of genomics. To date, he argues, the new topics of genomics governance have not been taken up adequately in the emerging institutional structures of policy-making. There exists a gap between policy challenges and the response. Gottweis highlights some of the problems of imbalance in technical knowledge between experts and publics, a recurrent theme of much of the recent social study of genetics. He also illustrates the ways in which socio-technical networks are often formed with unintended consequences.

Perhaps one of the most vivid examples of the importance of knowledge strategies in relation to genetics in recent years is the development of large-scale genetic databases in order to research the contribution of genes, lifestyle and environment to disease. Sometimes called biobanks or DNA banks or genetic databanks (Tutton and Corrigan 2004: 2), genetic databases raise many questions about governance, ethics and citizenship. Such databases may be extremely large, sometimes including the entire population (e.g. Icelandic Health Sector Database), and often include DNA, personal medical and genealogical data held over a very long period (ten years or more). The development of such databases, which often involve a substantial commitment of public resources, reflects belief in the public health benefits to be derived from genetic research. There has been a growing social science interest in the governmental and ethical challenges posed by such databases, especially around issues of informed consent and the security, ownership and use of collected information. For example, in 2004, an interdisciplinary group at the University of Vienna, under the direction of Herbert Gottweis, began an international study exploring a range of issues around biobanks and governance, including the extent to which biobank initiatives are indicative of a transformation in health policy, biomedical governance, and biopolitics. In a number of countries, concerns have been expressed about the adequacy of ethical protocols, about the security and value of collected information, and about the potential for commercial profiteering. In Britain, some of these and other concerns have been raised about UK Biobank (Petersen 2005). Concerns in the United Kingdom have centred on the possible misuse of samples, potential discrimination against disabled people, loss of participants' anonymity, profiteering by pharmaceutical and biotechnology companies, and employers and insurers gaining access to information and misusing it (Wellcome Trust & MRC 2000).

A number of questions can be raised in relation to genetic databases including: in what sense are they beneficial and who exactly benefits or is likely to benefit? What groups participate and do not participate, and why? How does the unique nature of genetic information, which is different from other kinds of health information by virtue of the fact that it is shared, influence notions of privacy and confidentiality? What role do genetic databases play, or are likely to play, in the wider processes of governance, and what can we learn from their emergence about conceptions of citizenship? To what extent, and how do genetic databases affect a transformation of identity, and what scope is there for individuals and groups to resist the implied 'geneticization' of health problems? How do regulatory frameworks serve to lend credibility and legitimacy to genetic databases? What specific new ethical and regulatory issues are raised by the long-term storage of genetic, medical and genealogical data, especially where commercial interests are involved?

Genetic databases depend heavily on the trust of publics that benefits will accrue in the future and that information will be secure and that privacy can be guaranteed. However, the involvement of the commercial sector in many, if not most, projects raises concerns about the privatization and commercialization of information that many people believe should be held in public hands and for public betterment, and about research being held hostage to market forces. So far, genetic databases have not been without their problems. In Iceland, monopoly control by DeCode over the country's health records and the Icelandic government's promise to provide the company with access to the nation's health records and assure them of the co-operation of its 270,000 population has caused considerable controversy (Pálsson and Rabinow 1999). In early 2004, the viability of the Icelandic project was questioned as a result of a case brought to Iceland's Supreme

Court by a citizen, who 'blocked the company from obtaining not just her health records but her dead father's because data in them could infringe her privacy' (McKie 2004: 2). The court ruled that the 1998 law that governs the country's database is unconstitutional because it fails to offer adequate personal privacy to participants (McKie 2004: 2). In Estonia, again in early 2004, the US backers of its genetic database, EGeen International, decided to delay a round of funding for the project until it established an agreement with the government on the project's priorities. The potential for citizen action and market responses such as these introduce an element of uncertainty about the longer-term viability of genetic databases and raise questions about the limits and failures of, and resistances to, governance through biopolitics. Research into the policies and practices supporting genetic databases and their operations, including practices of participant recruitment and the development of ethics and governance frameworks, can cast light on the broader workings of power, knowledge and politics and highlight the importance of the critical vantage point of view offered by governance and the governmentality perspective in particular.

The development of new genetic knowledge and technology has been accompanied by a burgeoning regulatory apparatus that reflects attempts at governance. Reports have been published by various authorities, including: national governments, the European Commission and WHO (see e.g. European Commission 2002; WHO 2002; Australian Law Reform Commission 2003; Human Genetics Commission 2000, 2002; UN report on genetically modified products 2004). Much of this 'governance' comprises regulatory policies and practices oriented to fulfilling specified objectives: stimulating development of, and engendering public confidence in, genetic technologies; advancing the dissemination and application of genetics knowledge within health services; and ensuring that genetics is applied for specified 'acceptable' purposes and does not produce 'deleterious' (by which is usually meant politically unacceptable) consequences. That is, governance is presented as activities or practices undertaken for the health and well-being of 'the public'. In our view, such 'governmental' efforts need to be seen in terms of broader workings of politics and power, and recognized for their intended and unintended effects; for example, the construction of populations, the reinforcement of inequalities and discrimination, and a heightening of risk awareness. Modern societies are characterized by the belief in rational science and rational administrative approaches to solving problems, especially problems created by new technological developments. Thus, activities concerning genetic research, and the provision and consumption of genetic knowledge, are seen as clearly definable and controllable, through techniques of classification, monitoring, and legislative action. 'Ethical' issues are seen as clearly delineable and governable through mechanisms such as protocols, ethics and governance frameworks, and ethics committees.

We have compiled this set of contributions to try to illustrate how the growing body of regulation and cross-sectoral initiatives that are being formed to govern the development of genomics is doing perhaps far more than is intended. We can see in these developments profound initiatives in the governance of society, of the public and the private domains, and of life itself. Foucault offers a useful set of ideas and questions in relation to genetics as it applies to public health and preventive medicine and a fruitful starting point for further study. This approach, at the very least, will guide study beyond the rather restricted focus on ELSI questions. We would caution against the use of Foucault's ideas alone in trying to provide understanding and critique of the range of issues of genetics and governance. Genetics constitutes a complex field of discourse and practice that requires interdisciplinary contributions and a range of methodologies. Moreover, Foucauldian scholarship is not without its own limitations, particularly when being used to contribute to radical politics of resistance or contestation (Petersen 2003b: 197–200). We would argue, however, that the potential substantial contributions of Foucauldian scholarship to understanding developments in genetics have not been widely recognized among scholars working on social aspects of genetics. The contributors in this volume have responded to our call for contributions in different ways, with a number drawing implicitly or explicitly on Foucault's ideas. We feel that they offer some ideas for addressing issues of governance and some provocation for future work of this kind.

References

Armstrong, D. (1983) *Political Anatomy of the Body: Medical Knowledge in Britain in the Twentieth Century*. Cambridge: Cambridge University Press.

Armstrong, D. (1995) 'The rise of surveillance medicine', *Sociology of Health and Illness*, 17: 393–404.

Australian Law Reform Commission (ALRC) and Australian Health Ethics Committee (AHEC) (2003) *Essentially Yours: The Protection of Genetic Information in Australia*. Canberra: ALRC and AHEC.

Bailey, R. (1996) 'Prenatal testing and the prevention of impairment: a woman's right to choose?' in J. Morris (ed.) *Encounters with Strangers: Feminism and Disability*. London: The Women's Press Ltd.

Beck-Gernsheim, E. (1995) *The Social Implications of Bioengineering*. Atlantic Highlands, NJ: Humanities Press.

Bunton, R. (1992) 'More than a woolly jumper: health promotion as social regulation', *Critical Public Health*, 3(2): 4–11.

Bunton, R., Nettleton, S. and Burrows, R. (eds) (1995) *The Sociology of Health Promotion: Consumption, Lifestyle and Risk*. London: Routledge.

Bunton, R. (1997) 'Popular health, advanced liberalism and Good Housekeeping Magazine' in Petersen, A. and Bunton, R. (eds) *Foucault, Health and Medicine*. London and New York: Routledge.

Burley, J. (ed.) (1999) *The Genetic Revolution and Human Rights: The Oxford Amnesty Lectures 1998*. Oxford: Oxford University Press.

Castel, R. (1991) 'From dangerousness to risk' in G. Burchell, C. Gordon and P. Miller (eds) *The Foucault Effect: Studies in Governmentality*. Hemel Hempstead: Harvester Wheatsheaf.

Chadwick, R., Levitt, M. and Shickle, D. (eds) (1997) *The Right to Know and the Right Not to Know*. Ashgate: Aldershot.

Dean, M. (1999) *Governmentality: Power and Rule in Modern Society*. London: Sage.

Duster, T. (2003) *Backdoor to Eugenics*. New York and London: Routledge.

Engelhardt, H.T. (2000) *The Philosophy of Medicine: Framing the Field*. Dordrecht: Kluwer Academic.

European Commission (2002) *Life Sciences and Biotechnology: A Strategy for Europe*. Luxembourg: Office for Official Publications of the European Communities.

Foucault, M. (1975) *The Birth of the Clinic: An Archaeology of Medical Perception*. New York: Vintage.

Foucault, M. (1980) *The History of Sexuality, Volume One: An Introduction*, trans. R. Hurley. New York: Vintage.

Foucault, M. (1990) *Care of the Self: History of Sexuality Vol 3*. Harmondsworth: Penguin.

Frank, A. and Jones, T. (2003) 'Bioethics and the later Foucault', *Journal of Medical Humanities*, 24(3/4): 179–186.

Fujimura, J.H. (2003) 'Future imaginaries: genome scientists as socio-cultural entrepreneurs', In A.H. Goodman, D. Heath and M.S. Lindee (eds) *Genetic Nature/Culture*, Berkeley, CA: University of California Press.

Fukuyama, F. (2003) *Our Posthuman Future: Consequences of the Biotechnology Revolution*. London: Profile.

Gastaldo, D. (1997) 'Is health education good for you?: Rethinking health education through the concept of bio-power', in A. Petersen and R. Bunton (eds) *Foucault, Health and Medicine*. London: Routledge.

Giddens, A. (1991) *Modernity and Self-Identity: Self and Society in the Late Modern Age*. Cambridge: Polity.

Ginsburg, N. (1998) 'Postmodernity and social Europe', in J. Carter (ed.) *Postmodernity and the Fragmentation of Welfare*. London: Routledge.

Gordon, C. (1991) 'Governmental rationality: an introduction', in G. Burchell, C. Gordon and P. Miller (eds) *The Foucault Effect: Studies in Governmentality*. Hemel Hemsptead: Harvester Wheatsheaf.

Habermas, J. (2003) *The Future of Human Nature*. Cambridge: Polity.

Haimes, E. (2002) 'What can the social sciences contribute to the study of ethics? Theoretical, empirical and substantive considerations', *Bioethics*, 16(2): 89–113.

Haraway, D. (1991) *Simians, Cyborgs, and Women: The Reinvention of Nature*. London: Free Association.

Hartouni, V. (1997) *Cultural Conceptions: On Reproductive Technologies and the Remaking of Life*. Minneapolis, MN: University of Minnesota Press.

Henderson, S. and Petersen, A. (eds) (2002) *Consuming Health: The Commodification of Health Care*. London: Routledge.

Hirst, P. (2000) 'Democracy and governance', in J. Pierre (ed.) *Debating Governance: Authority, Steering and Democracy*. Oxford: Oxford University Press.

Human Genetics Commission (HGC) (2000) *Whose Hands on your Genes? A*

Discussion Document on the Storage, Protection and Use of Personal Genetic Information. London: HGC.

Human Genetics Commission (HGC) (2002) *Inside Information: Balancing Interests in the Use of Personal Genetic Data. A Report of the Human Genetics Commission*. London: HGC.

Kickbusch, I. (2004) 'The end of public health as we know it: constructing global health in the 21st century, sustaining public health in a changing world', Vision to Action, World Federation of Public Health Associations (WFPHA), Tenth International Congress on Public Health, The Brighton Centre, Brighton, United Kingdom, 19–22 April.

Kjaer, A.M. (2004) *Governance*. Cambridge: Polity Press.

Latour, B. (1993) *We Have Never Been Modern*. Cambridge, MA: Harvard University Press.

Latour, B. (1987) *Science in Action*. Milton Keynes: Open University Press.

Lavis, J. and Sullivan, T. (1999) 'Governing health,' In D. Drache and T. Sullivan (eds) *Health Reform: Public Success, Private Failure*. London: Routledge.

Lemke, T. (2000) 'Neoliberalismus, Staat und Saelbsttechnologien. Ein Kritischer Überblick über die governmentality studies', *Politische Vierteljahresschrift*, 2 (In Press).

Lupton, D. (1999) *Risk*. London: Routledge.

Marteau, T. and Richards, M.P.M. (1996) *The Troubled Helix: Social and Psychological Implications of the New Human genetics*. Cambridge: Cambridge University Press.

McClean, S. (2004) 'Intergenerational justice' (commentary), *BioNews*, 240 (5–11 January): 1–3.

McKie, R. (2004) 'Icelandic DNA project hit by privacy storm', *Observer*, 16 May, http:www.guardian.co.uk/genes/article/0,2763,1217887,00.html (accessed 24 May 2004).

Malinowski, M.J. (1994) 'Coming into being: law, ethics, and the practice of prenatal genetic screening', *Hastings Law Journal*, 45(6): 1435–1526.

Nelkin, D. and Andrews, L. (1998) 'Homo economicus: commercialization of body tissue in the age of biotechnology', *Hastings Centre Report*, 28(5): 30–39.

Nettleton, S. 91997) 'Governing the Risky Self', in Petersen, A. and Buton, R. (eds), *Foucault, Health and Medicine*. London and New York: Routledge.

Novas, C. and Rose, N. (2000) 'Genetic risk and the birth of the somatic individual', *Economy and Society*, 29(4): 485–513.

O'Malley, P. (1996) 'Risk and Responsibility', in Barry, A., Osbourne, T. and Rose, N. (eds) *Foucault and Political Reason, Liberalism, Neo-liberalism and Rationalities of Government*. London: UCL Press.

Pálsson, G. and Rabinow, P. (1999) 'Iceland: the case of a national genome project', *Anthropology Today*, 15(5): 14–18.

Petersen, A. (1997) 'Risk, governance and the new public health', in A. Petersen and R. Bunton (eds) *Foucault, Health and Medicine*. London and New York: Routledge.

Petersen, A. (1999) 'Public health, the new genetics and subjectivity', in A. Petersen, I. Barns, J. Dudley and P. Harris, *Poststructuralism, Citizenship and Social Policy*. London: Routledge.

Petersen, A. (2003a) 'The new genetics and citizenship', Paper presented to Vital

Politics: Health, Medicine and Bioeconomics into the Twenty-First Century, London School of Economics, London, 5–7 September. http://www.lse.ac.uk/collections/BIOS/vital_politics_papers.htm (accessed 22 October 2004).

Petersen, A. (2003b) 'Governmentality, critical scholarship, and the medical humanities', *Journal of Medical Humanities*, 24(3/4): 187–201.

Petersen, A. (2005) 'Securing our genetic health: engendering trust in UK Biobank', *Sociology of Health and Illness*, 27(2): In press.

Petersen, A. and Bunton, R. (eds) (1997) *Foucault, Health and Medicine*. London and New York: Routledge.

Petersen, A. and Bunton, R. (2002) *The New Genetics and the Public's Health*. London: Routledge.

Petersen, A. and Lupton, D. (1996) *The New Public Health: Health and Self in the Age of Risk*. London: Allen and Unwin.

Rabinow, P. (1992) 'Artificiality and enlightenment: from sociobiology to biosociality', in J. Crary and S. Kwinter (eds) *Incorporations*. New York: Urzone.

Rheinberger, H-J. (2000) 'Beyond nature and culture: modes of reasoning in the age of molecular biology and medicine', in M. Lock, A. Young and A. Cambrosio (eds) *Living and Working with the New Medical Technologies*. Cambridge: Cambridge University Press.

Rhodes, R. (2002) 'Genetic links, family ties, and social bonds: rights and responsibilities in the face of genetic knowledge', in R. Sherlock and J. D. Morrey (eds) *Ethical Issues in Biotechnology*. Lanham, MD and Oxford: Rowman and Littlefield.

Rose, N. (1999) *Powers of Freedom: Reframing Political Thought*. Cambridge: Cambridge University Press.

Rose, N. (2001) 'The politics of life itself', *Theory, Culture and Society*, 18(6): 1–30.

Rosen, G. (1993[1958]) *A History of Public Health*. Baltimore, MD: Johns Hopkins University Press.

Rosenau, J.N. (1995) 'Governance in the 21st century', *Global Governance*, 1(1): 25–50.

Sample, I. (2004) 'Why limits must be set on the use of science', *Guardian*, 15 May, http:www.guardian.co.uk/genes/article/0,2763,1217443,00.html (accessed 24 May 2004).

Shakespeare, T. (1998) 'Choice and rights: eugenics, genetics and disability equality', *Disability and Society*, 13(5): 665–681.

Shakespeare, T. (2003) 'Rights, risks and responsibilities: new genetics and disabled people', in S. Williams, L. Birke and G.A. Bendelow (eds) *Debating Biology: Sociological Reflections on Health, Medicine and Society*. London: Routledge.

Tutton, R. and Corrigan, O. (2004) *Genetic Databases: Socio-Ethical Issues in the Collection and Use of DNA*. London: Routledge.

United Nations Food and Agriculture Organisation (FAO) 17 May 2004 'Agricultural Biotechnology: Meeting the Needs of the Poor?'

Wellcome Trust and MRC (2000) *Public Perceptions of the Collection of Human Biological Samples. Summary Report*, http://www.wellcome.ac.uk/en/genome/geneticsandsociety/hg16f002.html (accessed 22 October 2004).

Whitt, L.A. (1998) 'Biocolonialism and the commodification of knowledge', *Science as Culture*, 7(1): 35.

Wildavsky, A. (1988) *A Searching for Safety*. New Jersey: Transaction Publishers.

Williams, F. (2001) 'In and beyond New Labour: towards a new political ethics of care', *Critical Social Policy*, 27:467–493.

Williams, S.J., Birke, L. and Bendelow, G. (eds) (2003) *Debating Biology: Sociological Reflections on Health, Medicine and Society*. London: Routledge.

World Health Organization (1998) *Health 21 – Health for All in the 21st Century: An Introduction*, European Health for All Series no. 5. Copenhagen: WHO.

World Health Organization (2002) *Genomics and World Health*, Report of the Advisory Committee on Health Research. Geneva: WHO.

Part I

Ethics, risk and governance

Chapter 1

Ethics of clinical genetics

The spirit of the profession and trials of suitability from 1970 to 2000

Piia Jallinoja

Introduction

As research on and applications of human genetics expanded remarkably during the 1990s, claims that genetics and its applications should also be considered from an ethical viewpoint were increasingly raised. The background for the majority of ethical discussions and criticism was the argument that there is something special in the new genetics that requires particular attention (Williamson 1999).

This chapter examines those decades when medical ethics gradually became part and parcel of genetic testing, screening and counselling by analysing one institution founded in 1971 and three genetic counselling and screening programmes in the 1990s in Finland. In addition, text material written by Finnish physicians from 1970 to 2000 is analysed to determine the changes in the way ethics was argued for and materialized during three decades. The year 1970 is selected as a starting point for the analysis because during that year a liberal abortion law came into force and during the following years the organization of medical genetics services was activated. In 1971 the position of physician specialist in medical genetics was founded at the Family Federation of Finland, and in 1972 the first professorship in medical genetics in Finland was founded at the University of Helsinki (Kääriäinen 1991).

In the following, medical ethics is viewed from a sociological perspective (cf. Fox and DeVries 1998). This chapter examines the arguments and practices of medical ethics as part of a network of experts, codes, regulations and morals. Ethics is seen as an ongoing process tied up in the processes of medicine, legislation and the health care system. There is no single place or form for ethics in medicine; rather it is more or less intangible, occasionally verbalized as written codes, arguments or certain practices, and made concrete in the context of medical technologies. For example, the codes of ethics are here seen to further move into health care centres, screening projects and physician–patient interaction at genetic counselling (cf. Law and Singleton 2000).

To further define the scope of the sociology of ethics and the analysis of medico-ethical practice, I distinguish it from certain other views on medical ethics: I do not evaluate whether certain ethical principles have been obeyed in medical projects, nor do I offer suggestions for new ethical guidelines. Neither is ethics estimated in relation to some bioethical theory, by imposing a certain a priori definition of ethical principles on physicians' ethics (cf. Latour 1999a). Instead, this chapter treats the constructions and formulations of ethics and correctness presented in the study material as ways of dealing with and solving tensions caused by genetic screening. I examine the forms and contents of medical ethics: how ethics and the correctness of genetic screening were discussed and argued, and how and by whom the ethics was verified and especially how ethics was integrated into local medical research undertakings. Finally, I discuss what consequences these formulations of ethics carry with them. The formulations and execution of medical ethics are of central importance when analysing modern medical practice and health care systems.

Interviews and text data

This study is based on the analysis of interviews of health professionals and text material. Interviews were conducted within four projects related to genetic screening and counselling in Finland. Central professionals of the projects were contacted by phone. In all projects not only physicians were interviewed but psychologist or public health nurses were too. None of the persons contacted refused to be interviewed. The interviews were conducted for the most part at the office of the interviewee in Helsinki, Turku and Kuopio. The interviews, conducted from August 1997 to February 1998, lasted from 30 minutes to 2 hours and were tape-recorded and transcribed. For purposes of the present study, 11 interviews of physicians and psychologists were analysed. Although all these interviewees agreed that pseudonyms need not be used, I identify them here solely by their professional titles (for more detailed description of the interviews, see Jallinoja 2001).

Projects and institutions included in the study (project code in parentheses)

The diabetes screening project (D): in the Type 1 Diabetes Prediction and Prevention project, initiated in 1994, cord blood samples of newborns were screened for the presence of a gene related to susceptibility to diabetes. Those at increased genetic risk are followed-up for development of the first signs of diabetes. In cases where these occur, the child is included in a prevention trial that evaluates the efficacy of intranasal insulin in delaying or preventing diabetes onset.

The prenatal screening project (PS): in this project, gene tests for three gene defects were offered to all pregnant mothers at municipal maternity care centres in Kuopio during the years 1995 and 1996 (aspartylglucosaminuria (AGU), Fragile X and infantile neuronal ceroid lipofuscinosis (INCL)). During the mothers' first visit to the maternity care centre (between 8 and 12 gestational week) the public health nurses informed the mother about the tests and the disorders and distributed an information leaflet. During the next visit, the mother was asked whether she wanted to take the gene test. If she agreed, the blood sample for the carrier test was taken in the laboratory at the 13–15 week gestation period. If she tested positive, her partner was also offered a gene test. If the partner was also a carrier, amniocentesis was offered (see more in Jallinoja 2001).

Cancer counselling of the Finnish Cancer Associations (C): counselling for hereditary cancer was started in 1995 in regional cancer associations. The primary aim of the counselling was to clarify the situation in the family of the client by providing her or him information on cancer. Some of those seeking counselling may actually have a susceptibility to cancer and could thus be guided to appropriate follow-ups.

Genetic counselling at the Family Federation of Finland (FF): Family Federation of Finland is a non-governmental central organization in which the Department of Medical Genetics offers genetic counselling free of charge mainly for individuals and families seeking help.

In the interview extracts, the position or specialty of the interviewee is indicated as follows: physician or chief physician (*phys*) and psychologist (*psych*). If there are two interviewees with a similar position in the same project, the interviewees are numbered, e.g. physicians working in the diabetes project are referred to as *D/phys1* and *D/phys2*.

Text data consist of documents related to the projects listed above and include scientific, newspaper and magazine articles, leaflets, World Wide Web pages and official documents. In addition, text material from 1970 onwards was collected to further analyse the ethics of clinical genetics and gene research among Finnish physicians. First, booklets and manuals of medical ethics of the Finnish Medical Association (FMA; referred to as *Medical Ethics 1978*, etc.), including the Code of Medical Ethics of the FMA, were collected.

Second, articles of prominent physicians in the field of medical genetics in Finnish publications were collected. The prominent authors were determined as follows: an article search was conducted in MEDIC, the Finnish medical database (http://www.terkko.helsinki.fi/medic) that contains articles from 1978 onwards. The search was conducted with the keywords geeni*, geneett*, periytyvä, perinnöll* (gene*, genetic*, hereditary), genetic and hereditary in the two leading medical scientific journals in Finland, *Duodecim* and *Suomen Lääkärilehti*. The authors that resulted in at least five matches were classified as the prominent physician-authors in the field.

The authors were Leena Palotie, Albert de la Chapelle, Helena Kääriäinen, Pertti Aula, Kimmo Kontula and Reijo Norio, all of whom specialized in medical genetics. A new MEDIC search was performed in which all publications in MEDIC of these six authors were included, except congress abstracts, book chapters, obituaries, articles on issues outside genetics and heredity, articles on gene therapy and articles in languages other than Finnish or Swedish (the official languages in Finland). Journals other than *Duodecim* and *Suomen Lääkärilehti* were also included in order to scan the discussions in non-professional publications. To extend the research period to 1970, an additional article search was performed with Medline (does not include Finnish journals as extensively as MEDIC) for the six prominent authors. The total number of articles collected in this way was 105. References to the text data are in italics (e.g. *Aula 1970; Norio 1989* etc.).

'We have always been ethical': the spirit of the medical profession

For several interviewees, ethics had always been included in clinical genetics. For instance, both the former and the present chief physicians of the Family Federation saw ethics as something that had for almost three decades been the everyday topic in conversations at the clinic (*FF/phys1, FF/phys2;* also *Norio 1982*) even though the concept of ethics was not always mentioned (*FF/phys1*). The paediatrician of the Diabetes Project stated that in relation to the childhood diseases, ethical thinking and aspects had always been very predominant and clear (*D/phys1*). Likewise, the chief physician in the prenatal screening project considered that from the time when he started his career in obstetrics and gynaecology, the ethical principles of voluntariness and delivery of information were followed (*PS/phys*).

A closer analysis of the articles from the 1970s reveals that explicit references to medical ethics were very limited or non-existing *(Aula 1970; Aula et al. 1971*). In case the conditions for genetic counselling and prenatal diagnostics were discussed, it was noted that decisions regarding the offspring had always been left to the parents and would be based on the probability calculations provided by the genetic counselling (*Aula 1970;* also *Norio 1972*). Gene research and genetic counselling were also seen as methods of preventing disability and therefore as methods that saved money in treatment of 'the feebleminded' (*Norio 1970*).

The above-presented ethics was close to what Daniel Callahan has called the clinical ethics that refers to the day-to-day moral decision-making of those caring for patients, focusing on the individual case (Callahan 1995). Medical practice and medical ethics were interwoven and inseparable. Thus, ethical rules were seen to have their origins in practical experiences: certain practices were realized as advisable and some mistakes as fatal (*Medical Ethics 1978, 1980*). Clinical ethics is not a philosophical nor a theological

enterprise (Roy 1990, quoted in Reichlin 1994), but merely reflects the general spirit that inspires the profession (Spinsanti 1987, quoted in Reichlin 1994). This is the ethics that is seen as the age-old ways of practising proper medicine and helping the suffering patient, with 'head, hands and heart' as the chief physician of the Family Federation had expressed as the core of the matter (*Norio 1979*). It is the knowledge and conscience of a performer or an actor, and is close to professional ethics or professional etiquette, 'dignified spirit and good comradeship' as was expressed in the early twentieth century (Suomen Lääkäriliitto 1910–1985).

Although the notion of client and patient voluntary choice, privacy and provision of information were in some form present throughout the entire research period, it is clear that they become more strongly expressed in the articles of the late 1980s and the 1990s. The interviewees of the present study were asked to name characteristics of ethically approvable genetic counselling or screening projects. At the core of their estimations were autonomy, delivery of proper information, respect for privacy, honesty, beneficence and non-maleficence.

Medical theory, knowledge and experience as well as devoted attitude to treating and caring for patients as a package provided medical staff to a certain point with a flexible set of conventions for action in many situations (cf. Fujimura 1996). Although the above-described medical ethics still continued to be strongly present in 2000 (*Medical Ethics 2000*), it could no longer answer the increasing amount of new questions raised by growing potential for diagnosing hereditary diseases, especially prenatally.

The insoluble abortion question: a special case of medical ethics

Openness and ambiguity remained especially clear around the question of selective abortion, i.e. an abortion performed for certain undesirable disorders or diseases of the foetus. In the interviews – perhaps just because of this ambiguity – ethics was seldom connected with the question of abortion. One physician considered that in abortion issues 'one comes easily to a slippery ground . . . and in my opinion, it would take us all afternoon if we start to discuss those issues. It is better to stay apart [from the abortion issue]' (*FF/phys1*). For him, the issue of human worth of the foetus was difficult and insoluble (*Norio 1989*). Another physician considered that although there were no big ethical or legal questions, there might be on the individual and family levels 'serious ethico-moral critical situations that should be faced according to general principles of medical ethics and the conviction and hopes of the persons in question' (*Aula 1978*). Later he regarded selective abortion as a question related to a particular family, not a general question of medical ethics. Thus according to him, it was the living conditions of the parents that counted in selective abortion, not the severity of the disorder in question (*Aula 1988*). On the institutional level, abortion remained a contradictory issue (*Medical Ethics 1978, 1992, 2000*).

With respect to prenatal diagnostics, the duties of the physician were limited to technical procedures: taking the sample, estimating the risk of abnormality, evaluating the feasibilities and limits of prenatal diagnostics, providing the test results and estimating the situation with the family (*Medical Ethics 1992, 2000*). Decisions about tests and further measures were left to the pregnant woman, a position that was determined already in the abortion law of 1970. In the abortion question, the core of future formulations of medical ethics was already visible: the moral choices were up to the clients and further, the proper role of medical technology was to promote freedom of choice.

Operationalizing the spirit

Since the 1980s, and especially during the 1990s, the ethos of enthusiastic progress was clear in writings on genetics in Finnish medical journals, as it was in international publications. A great number of genetic diseases had been located, several genes and their mutations had been found, and although there were still many open medical questions and technical difficulties, development appeared to be rapid and the future promising (*Kere and de la Chapelle 1988; Kääriäinen, Palotie and Kontula 1994; Kääriäinen and Tryggvason 1995*). Methods for diagnosing disorders of the foetus increased significantly.

As medical genetics began to move increasingly from laboratories into clinical practice and even primary health care from the mid-1980s onwards, ethics was increasingly mentioned in medical articles as important. Usually, the ethics in the articles was limited only to a rather superficial flagging of the ethical questions, although some articles discussed ethical issues more extensively (e.g. *Aula 1988*; *Kääriäinen 2000*). In addition, an increasing number of ethical questions were specified, e.g. in relation to diagnostics of various diseases.

Furthermore, arguments about ethics began gradually to play a particular role in relation to the developing genetics. In ethics a general concern for the consequences of genetics was represented, a concern that did not necessarily mean a fundamental scepticism towards the whole of genetics. What was named as ethics cut across the other often-mentioned areas of concern, such as social, psychological and legal issues. Although ethics in academia was a discipline of its own, it also served as a viewpoint that almost everyone could have or even should have. Discussing medical ethics did not require special training.

Codes of ethics and ethics committees

Discussion of ethics was not limited only to the suggestive or general considerations or concerns, however. New sites and new forms for medical ethics

were developed. Ethics was formalized and institutionalized by physicians' associations and by public authorities governing medicine and health care. It was not left solely to the discretion of the physicians.

First, since the end of the Second World War, bioethics and medical ethics have increasingly taken the form of national and international ethical rules, codes and recommendations (Devettere 1995). In several European countries codes of ethics were published in the decade following the Nuremberg Code in 1947. After quieter decades, the publication increased in the late 1980s and 1990s (Herranz 1998). In 1956 the FMA adopted its first Code of Medical Ethics (Suomen Lääkäriliitto 1910–1985) and the following in 1988 (*Medical Ethics 1989*). In 1978, the FMA published its first booklet entitled *Medical Ethics* and its second edition was published in 1980. The first *Manual of Medical Ethics* of the Finnish Medical Association was published in 1989 (the following were published in 1992, 1996 and 2000). From the 1989 edition onwards the manuals included separate chapters on genetic counselling and prenatal diagnostics.

Second, during the late 1970s the National Board of Health recommended that all health care centres and hospitals should have ethics committees that would deal with research plans (Eettiset toimikunnat 1983). Finally, in 1999 a law came into force stating that all medical research plans must be evaluated and accepted in the ethics committee of the hospital district in question (Law on Medical Research 1999). Furthermore, the Working Group on Genetic Screening appointed by the Ministry of Social Affairs and Health recommended that an expert group guiding and evaluating genetic screening programmes and related social, ethical and legal issues should be established (Ministry of Social Affairs and Health 1998). In spring 2004, suggestions included in the memo were still waiting for further measures.

The aims of the research ethics committees were stated to be evaluation of the benefits, disadvantages and risks of research, as well as the content of information delivered to the research subjects (Wallgren 1986; *Medical Ethics 2000*), to guarantee the well-being and rights of research subjects (Idänpää-Heikkilä 1993) and assurance that the conditions defined in the Declaration of Helsinki and recommendation of the Council of Europe are realized in the research plan (Ministry of Social Affairs and Health 1992).

The importance of ethics committees was also acknowledged in the interviews carried out for the present research: the acceptance of the research plan in a local ethics committee was seen to reduce the ethical problems related to genetic screening (*PS/phys1*), and as a natural and important part of the research process (*D/phys1*). Thus, ethics committees governed for their part medical research. Unnecessary and badly conducted research was considered to be unethical (*Medical Ethics 2000*).

By the late 1990s a revival of medical ethics as a foundational spirit of the profession also occurred at the institutional level as exemplified by the reinstitution of voluntary swearing of the Physicians' Oath by graduating physicians in 1997 *Medical Ethics 2000*. In the 2000 edition of the Medical Ethics guidebook, the roots of medical ethics were highlighted. It was noted that the core of physicians' activity, its moral foundation is the same as it was during the time of primitive medicine (*Medical Ethics 2000*). The same trends have been reported to exist in the United States and United Kingdom since the 1960s (Nutton 1995).

'Let's sort this thing out!' Measuring ethicality

Several interviewees considered evaluation of psychological aspects related to genetic screening (*D/phys1*; *D/psych*) and of factors having impact on decision-making in regard to genetic counselling and screening (*C/psych*) to be part of ethics. As seen above, medical ethics was focused on patients' autonomy, choices and information. This view of medical ethics was taken as a starting point in the diabetes project (*D/psych; Simonen 1997*), prenatal screening project *(Ryynänen et al. 1999*) and cancer counselling project (*G/psych; C/phys1*) to measure the correctness or conduct of the projects. Opinions of Family Federation clients had also been evaluated during the 1980s and 1990s (*Somer et al. 1988; Järvinen et al. 1999).* As Ilpo Helén (2002) has noted in the United States and Great Britain, studies on 'psychological sequelae' in women subjected to prenatal testing and screening were conducted already in the late 1970s and 1980s.

The most rigorous psychosocial investigation was conducted in the diabetes project; it was also the largest undertaking of the research projects analysed here and was targeted on a significant public health problem. According to the project paediatrician, ethics consists of the practice of consent and understanding of how families accept the screening (*D/phys1*). For him it was not enough to discuss the ethics of gene technology and screening, instead they had to be tested, studied and sorted out. Accordingly, the participation rates and families' behaviour were constantly followed and analysed. This was the subproject in which psychologists were involved.

Thus, the satisfaction and participation of families were the realization of the often-repeated ethical principles – autonomy, privacy and informed consent. Ethics was equated with the approval of gene tests, attendance in screening and as the absence of severe psychological side-effects. Ethics was transformed into calculable definitions and statistical parameters that manifested the acceptability of screening. These measurements of acceptability matched with the overall statistical estimations of public health and incidences of gene defects among the population.

In the diabetes project the results on the acceptance and psychological reactions to the screening and gene test results were reported to 'support the continuation of screenings related to diabetes' (*Simonen 1997*). It was concluded that the satisfaction shown in participation suggests that positive test results did not cause harmfully strong worry in the families. Likewise, evaluation of the attendance rates and women's attitudes in the prenatal screening project showed 'the feasibility and acceptability of screening for fragile X mutations in low-risk pregnancies' (*Ryynänen et al. 1999*). Although ethics was not simply reduced only to these trails of approval, it constituted a viable argument in debates on genetic screening and testing during the late 1990s.

The formulations of medical ethics presented here may not be seen as hindrances to developments in medical genetics, but rather enabled its applications and served as guarantees of social, psychological and moral governability. These were formulations mainly of the medical profession: codes of ethics and ethics committees were in Finland mainly the domains of physicians, although some bioethicists and lawyers, for example, were included since the beginning (FMA 1975; Eettiset toimikunnat 1983). Furthermore, several interviewees noted that the psychosocial evaluations were initiated by the project physicians, not by experts in other disciplines (*D/phys1*; *D/psych*; *C/phys2; C/psych*). Since the 1970s especially, a few theologians and philosophers specialized in bioethics and were also to a certain extent included in the formation and discussions of medical ethics, although the institutionalization of bioethics was far less formal than in the United States, for example (Grodin 1995).

Discussion

In the course of the 1980s, controversies related to genetics were gradually articulated as questions of ethics. These were in turn further defined and governed by codes of ethics and ethics committees and integrated into measurements of attendance, approval and psychosocial consequences. Ethics, rules of proper conduct or ideas of good physicianship had been there all along, but in a more passive form, and were not constantly articulated or woven into various negotiations. Although the content or principles of ethics remained basically the same, from the 1980s onwards, ethics was more explicitly articulated and taken as an argument, as a tool in disputes and discussions on the new genetics.

Following Ulrich Beck, the situation may be interpreted as reflexive scientization *par excellence*, a process where the sciences are confronted by their own products, defects and secondary problems (Beck 1996). For Beck reflexive scientization is also characterized by the extension of scientific scepticism to the inherent foundations and external consequences of science itself. Although the physicians studied here were active in formalizing ethics and measuring the acceptance of their projects, the medico-ethical practices analysed in this chapter do not support Beck's suggestion about foundational scepticism. Indeed, Beck (1996) also points out that many sciences have taken up public criticism of themselves and transformed them into opportunities for expansion.

Ethics, however, was not an inevitable or absolute instrument for adjusting genetics into health care settings or remedy for frictions and insoluble questions. For example, some disability activists in Finland and elsewhere have seen the question of prenatal screening and selective abortion as a social or political question related to the disability community, not simply a question of individualized or case-based ethics (Könkkölä 1994; Shakespeare 1998).

Questions of genetic screening or selective abortion were not and are not presented, however, primarily as a disability rights or discrimination questions, but as questions of free, informed choice of the pregnant mother, family, client or patient. As Alan Petersen noted, efforts to expand genetic counselling services have occurred during a period in which citizens are increasingly expected to take greater responsibility for managing their own life and health (Petersen 1999). Indeed, genetics services are offered explicitly in the name of promoting informed choice (Petersen 1998; Chadwick 1999; Lippman 1999; Jallinoja 2001, 2002; Helén 2004).

Ethics aimed at balancing the formulated rights and freedoms of all actors involved and remained open to new situations. As Nikolas Rose (1999: 94–96) points out, this freedom and autonomy does not mean the absence of power. On the contrary, there are constant battles over freedom, over what it is, over what it should be and over what purports to be freedom while being its opposite. This, indeed, characterizes the negotiations over autonomous choice over gene tests and abortions. There is no 'naturally' occurring autonomy.

It is easy to see that medical ethics of medical genetics, in all its forms presented in this chapter, was in accordance with the above-described viewpoint of voluntary, informed choice. We should not stop, however, at these observations and explanations. There is more to be scrutinized, namely those circumstances in which the vague questions of ethics of screening, counselling and particularly of selective abortion were moulded and constituted anew into questions of suitability, functionality and non-maleficence. To understand the character and formulations of this new ethics, we should look more closely at certain characteristics of biosciences and medical ethics themselves as well as at certain new arrangements in physician–patient relationships.

First, during the three decades analysed here, the medical sphere was changed dramatically. Before the proliferation of prenatal screening technologies, the tasks of medical ethics were mainly about physician–patient relationship and about the collegiality among physicians. By the use of new prenatal diagnostics technologies a new actor – the foetus – was brought to the field of decision-making. The foetus had been there all along, but at the time when its features could not be effectively observed, speculations about its disorders were relatively weak and were not strongly connected with abortions. As Lorna Weir (1996) noted, the new prenatal diagnostic tests were distinctively different from prior forms of practice in that they were predictive at the individual level rather than being general statements about subpopulations. The foetus became a patient and an object of government (Weir 1996; see also Helén 2002, 2004). However, with new diagnostic methods, questions of the good life and limits of individuality became more intense and complicated. The foetus was at the same time diagnosable and human, but unable to express his or her will; the foetus was often both wanted and planned, but its life was tentative and conditional (see Rothman 1996). In addition, with the development of treatment of premature babies, the foetus could be during the same gestational week both kept alive if born prematurely or aborted due to severe disorder (STAKES 2000 – the National Research and Development Centre for Welfare and Health). Thus, as Thomas Lemke has expressed the situation, depending on the test results, the foetus would be legally enhanced and protected, or it would forfeit its legal status and mutate into foetal tissue (Lemke, unpublished observations). In obstetric care abortion has an ambivalent character: it is both a routine operation and an exception, 'an emergency solution' (Norio 2000). All in all, abortion in prenatal screening programmes is clearly a troublesome issue – the situation may be illustrated by the observation that in medical articles on prenatal screening for Fragile X, abortion is very seldom explicitly referred to (Jallinoja 2001).

Another major change that occurred during the research period was the increasing application of medical genetics in larger health care settings. Not only were rare gene defects investigated, but also the research had been more and more targeted on major public health problems, like cancer and diabetes. Thus, the number of actors involved in and affected by genetic technologies increased dramatically compared with the situation when only those families specifically concerned about hereditary disorders were the target group of genetic counselling. Interest groups, colleagues, health care staff, public health authorities, decision-makers and patients and clients had to be convinced about the beneficence and non-maleficence of genetic technologies.

Second, biosciences are relatively unarmed with respect to the new complicated situation, since they do not themselves carry the criteria for the 'good life' – other than healthy life. Healthy life as such, however, does not provide people with strong ethical arguments about good and bad, in the case of selective abortion or in knowing about one's susceptibility to some late-onset disease. It does not provide people with arguments about a good or satisfying life of parents or disabled children, whether knowledge about future illnesses increases happiness or not and what type of disorder in a child may become too heavy a burden for parents.

Third, in the old medical ethics there were neither mechanisms nor technologies to verify whether the encounter between physicians and patients is really ethically acceptable. Are the physicians and genetic counsellors really counselling according to informed consent? Are the clients truly free? Are the physicians' activities really in accordance with the principles written down in the manuals? Whereas it is relatively easy to calculate the incidence of gene defects, it is much more difficult to measure the incidence of ethically approvable actions.

In the above-described circumstances – a widening range of choices available both in personal conduct and in medical therapeutics – physicians' oaths, codes of ethics and various declarations provided some authority and standards (Nutton 1995). They provided some assurance that genetic counselling and testing practices were, at least in principle, in accordance with the same conditions wherever these practices appeared (cf. Timmermans et al. 1998).

Several authors have pointed to the appeal of quantitative measurement of opinions, aiming at scientific objectivity. Scientific objectivity has been seen to provide an answer to the moral demand for impartiality and fairness, do away with the idiosyncrasies of moral judgement (Porter 1995) and turn decisions into 'disinterested' ones (Rose 1999). On the other hand, Benjamin Ginsberg has noted that with a questionnaire study, public opinion is transformed from a spontaneous reaction to a constrained response, i.e. less disruptive and more amenable to governmental control (Ginsberg 1986; see also Rose 1999). Thus, medical ethics operationalized as acceptance of screening was the technology that provided medical staff with the means to evaluate and verify the actualization of voluntary choice and freedom, and consequently objectively argue in public, for example, about the acceptability of genetic screening. Following Latour (1999b), questionnaires made the invisible, intangible and weakly defined ethics visible, articulable and graspable and the local experiences of clients compatible with any experiences calculated by similar methods, but at the same time they moulded the concepts and contents of autonomy and choice.

During the late twentieth century, two types of practices coexisted. On the one hand, there was the day-to-day, experience-based medical ethics that had counselling of the concerned as its prime locus. On the other hand, there existed the operationalization of ethics in its various forms. Its prime loci were research projects, laboratories and large screening undertakings. In both practices the question of individuals' autonomous choice was central and subject to continuous disputes and negotiations.

Neither of these medico-ethical practices, however, provided the means to solve the moral dilemmas of selective abortion, good life, value of knowledge and control over one's life, that make the choices about tests and abortion for many so difficult. As soon as the contemplations of these dilemmas were expressed, they were pruned to individual's autonomous choice, attendance rates and clients' satisfaction, often manifested in questionnaire studies. Ethics, verified in these trials of suitability, leaves the moral decision for the self-reflexive individual.

Acknowledgements

This study received financial support from the Finnish Cultural Foundation, Jenny and Antti Wihuri Foundation, Doctoral Program of Public Health, Finland and the Doctoral Program of Sociology and Social Policy, University of Helsinki.

References

Aula, P. (1970) Periytyvien häiriöden intrauteriininen toteaminen. ***Duodecim****, 86, pp. 711–714.*

Aula, P., Karjalainen, O. & Leisti, J. (1971) Intrauteriinisesti diagnosoitu kromosomitranslokaatiotapaus. ***Duodecim****, 87, pp. 1372–1376.*

Aula, P. (1978) Periytyvien tautien ja kromosomihäiriöiden raskaudenaikainen toteaminen. ***Ketju****, nr. 1, pp. 19–23.*

Aula, P. (1988) Sikiödiagnostiikan eettisistä ongelmista. ***Kätilölehti****, 93/7, pp. 17–19.*

Beck, U. (1996) *The Risk Society: Towards a New Modernity*. London: Sage.

Callahan, D. (1995) 'Bioethics', in W. T. Reich (ed.) *Encyclopedia of Bioethics*. New York: Macmillan.

Chadwick, R. (1999) 'Genetics, choice and responsibility', *Health, Risk and Society*, 1(3): 293–300.

Devettere, R. (1995) 'The principled approach: principles, rules, and actions', in M. Grodin (ed.) *Meta Medical Ethics: The Philosophical Foundations of Bioethics*. Dordrecht: Kluwer Academic.

Eettiset toimikunnat. Toimintatietoja (Ethics committees. Information of activities) (1983) Helsinki: Lääkintöhallitus.

Finnish Medical Association (FMA) (1975) *Annual Report 1975*. Helsinki: FMA.

Fox, R. and DeVries, R. (1998) 'Afterword: the sociology of bioethics', in R. DeVries and J. Subedi (eds) *Bioethics and Society: Constructing the Ethical Enterprise*. Upper Saddle River, NJ: Prentice Hall.

Fujimura, J. (1996) *Crafting Science: A Sociohistory of the Quest for Genetics of Cancer*. Cambridge, MA: Harvard University Press.

Ginsberg, B. (1986) *The Captive Public: How Mass Opinion Promotes State Power*. New York: Basic Books.

Grodin, M. (1995) 'Introduction: the historical and philosophical roots of bioethics', in M. Grodin (ed.) *Meta Medical Ethics: The Philosophical Foundations of Bioethics*. Dordrecht: Kluwer Academic.

Helén, I. (2002) 'Risk and anxiety: polyvalence of ethics in high-tech antenatal care', *Critical Public Health*, 12(2): 119–137.

Helén, I. (2004) 'Technics over life: risk, ethics and the existential condition in high-tech antenatal care', *Economy and Society*, 33(1): 28–51.

Herranz, G. (1998) 'The inclusion of the ten principles of Nuremberg in professional codes of ethics: an international comparison', in U. Tröhler and S. Reiter-Theil (eds) *Ethics Codes in Medicine: Foundations and Achievements of Codification since 1947*. Aldershot: Ashgate.

Idänpää-Heikkilä, J. (1993) 'Eettiset toimikunnat tarvitsevat toimintaohjeet' (Ethics committees need guidelines), *Suomen Lääkärilehti*, 48(33): 3279–3281.

Jallinoja, P. (2001) 'Genetic screening at maternity care: preventive aims and voluntary choices', *Sociology of Health & Illness*, 23(3): 286–307.

Jallinoja, P. (2002) *Genetics, Negotiated Ethics and the Ambiguities of Moral Choices*. Helsinki: National Public Health Institute.

Järvinen, O., Aalto, A.-M., Lehesjoki, A.-E., Lindlöf, M., Söderling, I., Uutela, A. & Kääriäinen, H. (1999) Carrier testing of children for two X linked diseases in a family based setting: a retrospective long term psychosocial evaluation. ***Journal of Medical Genetics****, 36, pp. 615–620.*

Kääriäinen, H. (1991) 'Perinnöllisyysneuvonnan uranuurtajana' (The pioneer of genetic counselling), in *Väestöliitto 1941–1991. Perheen puolesta*. Helsinki: Family Federation of Finland.

Kääriäinen, H., Palotie, L. & Kontula, K. (1994) Suomalaiset geenit ja niiden tutkiminen. ***Duodecim****, 110, pp. 639–40.*

Kääriäinen, H. & Tryggvason, K. (1995) Perinnölliset munuaistaudit ja niiden geenidiagnostiikka. ***Duodecim****, 111, pp. 1398–1400.*

Kääriäinen, H. (2000) Geenitekniikan lupaukset ja uhkakuvat. ***Duodecim****, 114, pp. 2461–4.*

Kere, J. & de la Chapelle, A. (1988) Geenikartoituksen uudet menetelmät. ***Duodecim****, 104, pp. 1439–1447.*

Könkkölä, K. (1994) 'Vammaisuus ei ole taakka' (Disability is not a burden), *Kynnys* 1994; 3: 8–9.

Latour, B. (1999a) 'On recalling ANT', in J. Law and J. Hassard (eds) *Actor Network and After*. Oxford: Blackwell and The Sociological Review.

Latour, B. (1999b) *Pandora's Hope: Essays on the Reality of Science Studies*. Cambridge, MA: Harvard University Press.

Law, J. and Singleton, V. (2000) 'This is not an object', (draft) published by the Centre for Social Science Studies and the Department of Sociology, Lancaster University, http://www.lancaster.ac.uk/sociology/soc032jl.html (accessed 29 March 2000).

Law on Medical Research (1999) Dnro: 488/1999. http://www.finlex.fi

Lippman, A. (1999) 'Choice as a risk to women's health', *Health, Risk & Society*, 1(3): 281–291.

Medical Ethics. Lääkärin etiikka. *(1978) Helsinki: Suomen Lääkäriliitto.*

Medical Ethics. Lääkärin etiikka. *(1980) Helsinki: Suomen Lääkäriliitto.*

Medical Ethics. Lääkärin etiikka. *(1989) Helsinki: Suomen Lääkäriliitto.*

Medical Ethics. Lääkärin etiikka. *(1992) Helsinki: Suomen Lääkäriliitto.*

Medical Ethics. Lääkärin etiikka. *(1996) Helsinki: Suomen Lääkäriliitto.*

Medical Ethics. Lääkärin etiikka. *(2000) Helsinki: Suomen Lääkäriliitto.*

Ministry of Social Affairs and Health (1992) *Eettisen toimikuntien toiminta* (Activities of ethics committees). Letter. Dnro 2899/09/92.

Ministry of Social Affairs and Health (1998) *Geeniseulontatyöryhmän muistio* (Workgroup of genetic screening: a memo). Helsinki: Ministry of Social Affairs and Health.

Norio, R. (1970) Vajaamielisyys käytännön ongelmana. ***Kätilölehti****, 75, pp. 467–475.*

Norio, R. (1972) Kliinikon genetiikka. ***Duodecim****, 88, pp. 15–23.*

Norio, R. (1979) Lihassairaudet perinnöllisinä tauteina. ***Duodecim****, 95, pp.*

1468–1473.

Norio, R. (1982) Perinnöllisyys ja vammaisuuden ennalta ehkäisy. ***CP-lehti,*** *17/8, pp. 2–3.*

Norio, R. (1989) Onko sikiö ihminen. ***Suomen Lääkäfilehti,*** *44, pp. 3279–80.*

Norio, R. (2000) *Suomi-neidon geenit* (Genes of Maiden Finland). Helsinki: Otava.

Nutton, V. (1995) 'What's in an oath?', *Journal of the Royal College of Physicians of London*, 29(6): 518–524.

Petersen, A. (1998) 'The new genetics and the politics of public health', *Critical Public Health*, 8(1): 59–71.

Petersen, A. (1999) 'Counselling the genetically "at risk": the poetics and politics of "non-directiveness"', *Health, Risk & Society*, 1(3): 253–265.

Porter, T. (1995) *Trust in Numbers: The Pursuit of Objectivity in Science and Public Life*. Princeton, NJ: Princeton University Press.

Reichlin, M. (1994) 'Observations on the epistemiological status of bioethics', *Journal of Medicine and Philosophy*, 19(1): 79–102.

Rose, N. (1999) *Powers of Freedom: Reframing Political Thought*. Cambridge: Cambridge University Press.

Rothman, B.K. (1996) *The Tentative Pregnancy: Amniocentesis and the Sexual Politics of Motherhood*. London: Pandora and HarperCollins.

Roy, D. (1990) 'Orientamenti etendenze della bioetica nel ventennio 1970–1990', in C. Viafora (ed) *Vent'anni di bioetica*. Fondazione Lanza Gregorianna Libreria Editrice, Padova. p 93–122.

Ryynänen, M., Heinonen, S., Makkonen, M., Kajanoja, E., Mannermaa, A. & Kirkinen, P. (1999) Feasibility and acceptance of screening for fragile X mutation in low-risk pregnancies. ***European Journal of Human Genetics,*** *7, pp. 212–216.*

Shakespeare, T. (1998) 'Choices and rights: eugenics, genetics and disability equality', *Disability & Society*, 13(5): 665–681.

Simonen, P. (1997) ***Lapsen diabetesalttius ja perhe.*** *[Child's susceptibility to diabetes and the family] University of Turku, Department of Psychology, licentiate's dissertation.*

Somer, M., Mustonen, H. & Norio, R. (1988) Evaluation of genetic counselling: recall of information, post-counselling reproduction, and attitudes of the counsellees. ***Clinical Genetics,*** *34, pp. 352–365.*

Spinsanti, S. (1987) *Etica bio-medica*. Paoline, Cinisello Balsamo.

STAKES (2000) *Birth Register 1991–1995*. Helsinki: National Research and Development Centre for Welfare and Health.

Suomen Lääkäriliitto 1910–1985 (1985) Helsinki: Suomen Lääkäriliitto.

Timmermans, S., Bowker, G. and Star, S.L. (1998) 'The architecture of difference: visibility, control, and comparability in building a nursing interventions classification', in M. Berg and A. Mol (eds) *Differences in Medicine*. Durham, NC: Duke University Press.

Weir, L. (1996) 'Recent developments in the government of pregnancy', *Economy and Society*, 25(3): 372–392.

Wallgren, E. (1986) Eettiset toimikunnat. *Suomen Lääkärilehti*, 41: 1594–1595.

Williamson, R. (1999) 'What's 'new' about genetics'? *Journal of Medical Ethics*, 25: 75–76.

Chapter 2

Risk management and ethics in high-tech antenatal care

The Finnish experience

Ilpo Helén

Introduction

The subject of this chapter is the abortion problems brought about by advanced techniques of foetal diagnosis and antenatal screening (including genetic testing) in maternity care. 'Selective abortion', as the operation is called in professional circles, is a prime example of the type of ethical problem in high-tech medicine highlighted by the feminist critique of new reproductive medicine (e.g. Overall 1987; Hubbard 1990; Rothman 1996) and the discussion on the geneticization of medicine (e.g. Lippman 1991; Cowan 1993; Lemke 2000).

This new abortion question exemplifies the ways in which problems involved in the implementation of high-tech biomedicine in clinical practice and primary health care are defined *ethical*. Furthermore, selective abortion and the related ethical controversies are embedded in the emerging forms of bio-power, or *vital politics* (Rose 2001; see also Lemke 2000: 259–269). The latter is closely connected to the unforeseeable opportunities to mould human bodies and life that have been opened by the rapid development of medical technology, especially the expansion of molecular genetics in medicine (e.g. Flower and Heath 1993; Rabinow 1996; Lemke 2000; Helén 2004b). Characteristic is the tendency to think in terms of risk and to emphasize health and 'life itself' as matters of individuality and selfhood (Novas and Rose 2000; Rose 2001; Helén 2004a).

As is well known, the technological 'imperative' and risk rationality impose changes throughout Western health care, including public health. Not only are practices and policy-making challenged, but also the very concepts of health and illness and the objectives of medicine are liable to transformation (e.g. Yoxen 1984; Rheinberger 1995; Petersen 1998; Koch 1999; Helén 2004b). Moreover, underlying controversies in Western medicine, such as the tensions between clinical and laboratory medicine and between primary and specialized health care, are aggravated. In particular, extension of the scope of preventive health control and the idea of health risks have served to deepen the rift between rapid advances in diagnostics and minor progress in therapeutics, a claim well exemplified by developments in medical genetics (Rheinberger 1995; Rabinow 1996; Koch 1999).

The definition of selective abortion as an ethical problem is related to the tensions engendered by the implementation of advanced medical technology and the process of change thus set in motion. When foetal diagnosis and antenatal screening are disputed in terms of ethics, a thought-space around the 'ethical issues' is unfolded in which the above discords can be attempted to reconcile. In this chapter, I take a closer look at this thought-space and its groundwork. I distinguish different settings in which the questions of foetal diagnosis are defined as the ethical ones, arguing that the ethical problem varies from one context of 'ethicalization' to another.

First, I present the Finnish case, on which my study is based. I then discuss the role of risk information in carrying out foetal diagnosis and antenatal screening. From there, I proceed to analyse the meaning of 'ethics' in relation to foetal diagnosis in general and to the principle of informed consent. The next section forms the core of my inquiry. In it, I study individualized risk, the existential situation it imposes, and the related discourse and practice of anxiety management. I conclude my chapter with a general remark on 'ethicalization' of current biomedical technology.

The Finnish case

My study is based on an analysis of the discourse on the implementation of high-tech foetal diagnosis and antenatal screening in Finnish maternity care.[1] Due to the particular characteristics of Finland's maternity care system, the case study highlights the implementation of advanced medical technology as a public health matter.

Maternity care in Finland follows the Nordic model of public health and welfare services. Based on public funding and provision of facilities, it is guided by the principle of equal and universal accessibility. At the heart of the system are maternity care centres, funded and run by the municipalities. Nowadays, they are usually integrated with municipal health care centres. The maternity care centre provides check-ups of pregnant women by a public health nurse or midwife and routine health examinations by a physician, and it seeks to provide women with psychosocial care and advice about caring for their babies. The centres also carry out routine ultrasound scan examinations. The service is available free of charge to every pregnant woman. Moreover, a pregnant woman has to attend a maternity care centre in order to be eligible for social maternity benefits. Not surprisingly, then, practically every pregnant women in Finland makes use of the public maternity care system (Gissler et al. 1996; STAKES 1996).

Maternity care centres are integrated with public hospitals, in larger towns also with university hospitals. Obstetrical and gynaecological clinics in hospitals provide expert consultation to the centres, perform high-tech antenatal tests and diagnoses and see to the medical care of high-risk pregnancies. Birth care likewise comes within the domain of public hospitals (in fact, almost all deliveries occur in them), and they also carry out abortions (STAKES 1996).

Finland's abortion policy, like maternity care, is characteristically Nordic. It is a combination of legislation that acknowledges abortion as the woman's personal choice and a controlling practice that attempts to keep the number of abortions 'acceptable' by means of contraceptive and sexual education and frequent follow-ups by public health authorities. The entitlement to terminate pregnancies rests largely with public hospitals (Helén and Yesilova 2003: 245–248).

The liberal abortion policy since the early 1970s implies unreserved approval of abortion on the basis of foetal diagnosis. The Abortion Act 1970 states that a pregnancy may be terminated 'if there is reason to assume that the child would be mentally deficient or would have or develop severe illness or malformation'. In 1986, the limit for legal abortion based on this indication was extended from the twentieth to the twenty-fourth gestational week. Annually, some 200 pregnancies are terminated due to 'foetal indication'; the total number of abortions, however, exceeds 10,000 (Eronen et al. 2003).

The implementation of advanced techniques for foetal diagnosis and screening in Finnish maternity care exemplifies the major change of Western antenatal care since the late 1960s. The definition of pregnancy in terms of risk and the increasing emphasis on specific 'risk factor' assessment by advanced technology, the emergence of predictive diagnostic control of the *foetus* as a task at least as important as the health care of pregnant women (Oakley 1993: 65–77; Weir 1996; Ruhl 1999) and the tendency to shift the focus from primary health care units to specialized hospital and laboratory facilities (e.g. Oakley 1993: 189–197) are traits that are pre-eminent in the development of Finnish antenatal care during the 1980s and 1990s (Hemminki et al. 1990; Wrede 1997). The major innovative techniques of foetal diagnosis and testing were introduced in Finland as soon as they became technically available. The ultrasound scan to detect foetal malformations and developmental disorders was tested in maternity care in the early 1970s. Today over 90 per cent of municipalities offer the scan to all pregnant women as a part of routine prenatal medical examinations. Amniocentesis and chorionic villus sampling (CVS) for detecting chromosomal abnormalities were introduced into obstetrical practice in the mid-1970s. In the late 1970s and early 1980s, local pilot projects were launched to screen congenital nephrosis of the Finnish type by a predictive maternal serum alpha-fetoprotein blood test, combined with amniocentesis or CVS as a diagnostic test. Local experiments to screen pregnant women aged 35 or over by a combination of maternal serum blood sample tests and amniocentesis or CVS to detect the chromosomal disorder causing Down syndrome were launched in the late 1980s. By the mid-1990s, the above test kit was an integrated part of the maternity care of that age group in two-thirds of municipalities, although the technique has increasingly been replaced by the ultrasound screening of Down syndrome at the turn of the 2000s. The screening procedures are carried out at the specialist clinics and laboratories in public district hospitals or university hospitals (Asmala 1995; Santalahti and Hemminki 1998).

Thus, antenatal screenings have been firmly established in Finnish maternity care, and this development engendered bright prospects for experimentation of medical genetics in primary health care. Strikingly, the introduction of DNA-based testing in maternity care has been quite self-evidently considered as just a continuation of the 'improvement' of antenatal care by advanced technology in Finland (see Ettorre 1996). This is well illustrated by the statement of two prominent medical geneticists:

> The organization of foetal diagnosis has functioned successfully for almost twenty years, and it has established a proper infrastructure that connects maternity care centres, units of clinical genetics and chromosomal laboratories. Genetic screenings should be carried out in a similar manner, within the framework of the primary health care system.
>
> (Aula and Leisti 1994: 754. Translation IH)

The recommendation was put into practice in a few local experiments in the early 1990s. At that time, a foetal DNA test for aspartylglucosaminuria, Fragile X syndrome and infantile neuronal ceroid lipofuscinosis became technically available for clinical use (see Syvänen et al. 1992), and women receiving maternity care were screened by this test in some municipalities. The trials were part of an ongoing effort to introduce medical genetics into clinical practice, the objective being to investigate the potential of DNA-based testing and genetic counselling in screening groups and families at risk for a particular genetic disease. Many Finnish geneticists, especially in the early 1990s, were convinced of the benefits and success of large-scale genetic screening. They were encouraged by studies in genetic epidemiology showing the unique genetic composition of the Finnish population, with its high frequency of certain rare monogenetic diseases, known collectively as 'the Finnish disease heritage', and the almost total absence of cystic fibrosis and phenylketonuria (PKU) (e.g. Chapelle 1993). However, genetic screenings have not been established permanently in Finnish maternity care; in fact, any similar experiment has not been launched since the mid-1990s, partly due to the shift in focus of Finnish medical genetics from rare monogenetic diseases to common diseases like asthma and diabetes.

Nevertheless, this endeavour on genetic screening is significant because it highlights the close relationship between the institutions of medical science and public health care in Finland. This proximity is crucial in the implementation of new knowledge and techniques in medical practice, because it gives biomedical science a particularly influential status in public health in Finland. Furthermore, certain features of the Finnish debate over policy-making on advanced techniques of foetal diagnosis in maternity care were highlighted in these experiments. Most importantly, problems and issues involved in the implementation of new technology together with the demand for a more broadly based discussion of the subject are mostly brought up by medical experts and public health authorities (see Jallinoja 2001, 2002). The role of critical lay movements and discourses has been suprisingly marginal. Consequently, questions on the subjection of pregnant women to new medical technology and the potential increase in discrimination against disabled people have been articulated as topics of policy-making, not as political issues raised by any organized political movement. Thus, in Finland, due to the typically Nordic emphasis on the public nature of health care, controversial issues of advanced medical technology are readily defined as public health matters, but they appear as problems to be solved rather than issues to be disputed. All in all, Finnish discussion and policy-making have focused on problems concerning the antenatal screening of a population or certain population groups; issues related to the availability of advanced antenatal diagnostic testing and genetic counselling have attracted little attention.

Risk and the ethics of informing

The knowledge provided by foetal diagnosis tells us primarily about the probability of future illness and disease, thus epitomizing the *predictive* nature of today's high-tech medicine (see Kevles 1993: 30–32; Koch 1999). The idea of *risk* is indispensable to the functioning of such medical practice, since it provides a form, albeit equivocal, for reasoning, discourse and the ordering of reality. Through risk, the relationship between individuals and the population has been reassembled in terms of potentiality and probability, and is now conceived of as varying clusters of calculable 'risk factors'. Moreover, the idea of risk implies activity, since it facilitates the transfiguration of dangers into definable, even calculable 'objects' that can be acted upon. Thus it moulds the perspective of the future from a state of waiting to decision and action. Finally, risk is polyvalent. The definition, uses and implications of risk vary from one context to another. (For an overview of discussions on risk, see Baker and Simon 2002; Garland 2003.)

The latter aspect of risk is particularly relevant to the implementation of high-tech reproductive medicine. As mentioned, knowledge of the risk related to pregnancy, the foetus or some other 'factor' of the medical condition is constitutive of contemporary medical maternity care (Wrede 1997; Ruhl 1999). However, knowledge of risk and even the figure of risk are not unambiguous. The epistemic, technical and practical definitions of risk and the implications of risk for the health of a population differ from those relevant in clinical and health care practice. The meaning of risk is different again in situations where pregnant women have to make personal decisions concerning screening and diagnostic testing. A kind of oscillation between *group risk* and *clinical risk* characterizes antenatal screening procedures and foetal diagnosis in maternity care. The former is defined epidemiologically and indicates the risk faced by a pregnant woman on the basis of her belonging to a certain risk population. The latter is rendered by a diagnostic operation or test indicating potential abnormality in the life process of a pregnant woman or in the foetus (see Weir 1996). Furthermore, in the case of amniocentesis and CVS, these advanced techniques in themselves carry a *technical risk* of causing miscarriage.

Information on risks has acquired a central role in high-tech antenatal care. This information is supposed to translate group, clinical or technical risks into a form that enables pregnant women to assess the dangers and decide personally whether or not they should undertake the procedures of screening or testing (see Lemke 2000: 251–254; Rapp 2000: 63–73). The 'ethical' problems engendered by the implementation of high-tech reproductive medicine in clinical practice and primary health care focus very closely on questions of risk informing. They appear complicated and profound because they are closely related to clinical practices and the conduct of personnel. A core issue is the linkage of advanced antenatal diagnostics to selective abortion. The controversies have become particularly critical with regard to Down syndrome screening. Also a genetic screening experiment in Kuopio in the mid-1990s raised a debate on ethical problems and was eventually suspended because of this (Jallinoja 2001).

Palpably, knowledge of risk is at the heart of the problem and controversy, especially in the Kuopio case. The issue, however, is not one of truthfulness or technical appropriateness of knowledge of the diseases mentioned; rather, it is the use and worth of such knowledge as *information* on genetic risks and antenatal screening procedures that is shared with women attending the maternity clinic (see Lemke 2000: 251–254). In other words, the paramount ethical problem concerns the *value* of the knowledge of risk and probability provided by high-tech predictive diagnosis. The questions are: is it good to know in advance; does knowing that one is at risk bring any benefit and happiness; or does such knowing merely cause distress and grief to those subjected to it?

Regarding advanced foetal diagnosis, antenatal screenings and selective abortion, the problem of the value of risk information is discerned as ethical in three settings. First, there is the discourse on the *general* moral and social consequences of the application of new technology, reflecting contemporary abstract discussion on bioethics. This is marked by the attempt to find a kind of minimum of 'sacredness' on which to base the ethical code of biomedicine that respects the sanctity of life and the rights and dignity of individuals (e.g. Dworkin 2001). Further, general ethical problems are related to 'social implications'. The main issues are whether expansion of antenatal screening and testing will lead to increasing discrimination against disabled and sick people in different fields of society, and whether women's control over their own bodies will be subverted. The line of moral reasoning focusing on general ideas of respect for life, human dignity and social equality has been influential in policy-making and in processes defining guidelines for antenatal screening and diagnostic testing, led by physicians and public health authorities (Jallinoja 2002: 108–110).

Second, this discourse on the general ethical problems involved in foetal diagnosis is embedded in another, more specific, setting. At the heart of this is the practical rationale according to which use of state-of-the-art foetal diagnostics in maternity care becomes possible and appropriate. It puts the pregnant woman (and her family) in a key position in the execution of this array of medical operations. In essence, this logic is an attempt to reconcile the demands of advances in biomedical science with the principle of the autonomy of the person subjected to medical treatment. This liberal principle has two different contexts of articulation. One is the medical ethics originating in the Nuremberg Code, introduced in 1947, that emphasizes the patient's right of choice and consent with regard to any medical examination or operation (Faden and Beauchamp 1986: 86–99, 152–167). The other is the idea that women have a personal right to rule their own bodies and make reproductive choices, as advocated ardently by feminist movements since the late 1960s and acknowledged in contemporary liberal abortion legislation (e.g. Luker 1985).

The basic rationale of reconciliation is simple. Power over decisions regarding antenatal medical operations has been divided, the field of action of the medical profession being restricted to technical and controlling operations. Accordingly, the actual performance of screening and diagnostic procedures, and also of abortion, has been entrusted to maternity care centres, laboratories and specialist medical clinics. Moreover, the power to carry out these procedures is in a sense also split. The public health authorities, in consensus with authorities in medical science, set guidelines that define which antenatal screening and diagnostic techniques can be used as routine procedures and which should be reserved for special risk groups. However, both the 'ethical' discourse and the practical guidelines underline repeatedly that, in individual cases, the excecution of any procedure – screening, diagnostic testing or, especially, abortion – should be based on the personal judgement and decision of a pregnant woman who has received 'adequate' and 'non-directive' information about the procedure in question. As many studies suggest, such an emphasis could be seen to imply that the *informed consent* of the patient is considered as a constitutive *ethical* requirement for the high-tech management of pregnancy (Faden 1991; Koch and Stemerding 1994: 1217–1218; Petersen 1999: 255–258).

Medical knowledge of risk as *information* given by the maternity care machinery to the pregnant woman to be tested or screened plays thus a key position in safeguarding the ethical acceptability of foetal diagnosis and screening procedures. The functioning of advanced antenatal testing and screening is based on the assumption that 'mothers' (with their families) are capable, on the basis of proper information, of making a choice whether or not to participate in the tests and, in the event of findings indicating abnormality of the foetus, whether or not to have an abortion. Thus, medical risk management creates a situation where the machinery of reproductive health care leaves the decision-making concerning any procedure to the pregnant woman. It withdraws to a position in which its responsibility is purely *technical*: it only exposes the health risks involved in a pregnancy or indicated by findings of foetal diagnosis. The *ethical* responsibility lies with 'the mother'.

Risk individualized

This split brings us to the third setting. In it, selective abortion actually enters the agenda of the ethical discussion on high-tech reproductive medicine. Remarkably, policy-makers and spokespersons of the medical and public health professions consider that this facet of the issue belongs outside their sphere of judgement, since the decisions at stake are depicted as solely intimate matters and personal choices. This view applies especially to selective abortion. In fact, the physicians involved in experimenting with and using advanced methods of antenatal screening and diagnosis are rather reluctant to plumb the profound problems involved in abortion (Jallinoja 2002: 108), as is reflected even in the Finnish public health guidelines for antenatal screenings (STAKES 1995, 1999; Ministry of Social Affairs and Health (MSH) 1998). This reluctance further stresses that pregnant women receiving maternity care are *subjectivized* as choosing and consenting individuals by the practices of high-tech reproductive medicine.

Consequently, the ethical question of high-tech antenatal care is intensified in situations in which pregnant women make personal decisions about participating in screenings and foetal diagnosis. When a pregnant woman considers her consent, parameters indicating the health risk of the foetus and risks in the diagnostic test obviously come to the fore. However, the situation demands her to be a subject of choice, which goes beyond the calculation of risks.

Becoming a subject of choice requires the pregnant woman to analyse and work through her aspirations and feelings related to having a child and, indeed, her own life as a whole. First, she has to decide if she wants to have the knowledge provided by chromosomal or DNA-based tests. She also has to deal with her desire to acquire information, and thus 'be assured', about the health of her baby. Second, she has to think about whether or not she will have an abortion on the basis of 'foetal indication'. This leads to complicated considerations. The pregnant woman has to envision the possible life course of her would-be child and, in relation to this, anticipate her own life in future. Third, she has to reflect on herself as a person making a choice and think through questions of selfishness, responsibility, sacrifice, suffering, guilt, etc. (Rothman 1996: 49–85; Rapp 2000: 129–142, 223–240, 251–253). These intimate considerations form the very foundation of the woman's decisions concerning procedures of high-tech antenatal diagnosis, implying that the focus of consent and choice is the person's relation to the self and personal life.

Hence, bioethics of high-tech reproductive medicine is *formally* based on the idea of the moral autonomy of the individual, represented by the principles of informed consent and woman's choice. However, the *content* of bioethics is tied up with reflections on the relation to the self, that is, to problematization and the shaping of oneself as a moral subject (see Foucault 1985: 25–32). Hence, the particular situations in which pregnant women as particular individuals make reproductive choices are constitutive for the ethics of contemporary high-tech antenatal care. Accordingly, an effective code of moral conduct and responsibility that would bear on every woman's choice is hardly conceivable. Thus, *ethics is not generalizable but dispersed.*

The high-tech machinery of reproductive medicine displays the multiplicity, randomness and uncertainty of life 'itself' to the pregnant woman, affords her means to influence her own destiny and the life of her child, and compels her to make a choice. By doing so, it imposes an *existential* condition. In other words, the pregnant woman is put into a situation in which her choice and personal responsibility can be adequately described in terms of existentialist philosophy.[2] There is a basic tension between the uncertainty of life and definite personal choice. The outcome of choice is open and may lead to exceptional and undesired deeds such as abortion. Moreover, the pregnant woman as a responsible person has to make the choice solely on the basis of her own life and situation, without appealing to any transcendental principle or instance. As a result, the self becomes the dominant anchor point of the choice. In fact, ethics and responsibility are articulated through the idea that the choice essentially concerns the nature and qualities of the self, a conception that implies a certain solitude in making a choice on a matter of life and death. Yet, the foetus as 'the other', whose life is fundamentally influenced by the choice, is involved in the situation, too. The personal choice is indispensably related to, although not determined by, 'the other'. When a person makes a choice focused on her own life, destiny and the self, her own existence becomes involved in and opens up towards the existence of 'the other'. Ultimately, existential responsibility, with all its weight, originates in this involvement.

However, this existential condition is unusual since it is embedded in and even imposed by advanced medical technology. The peculiarity is epitomized in the form of 'the other', shaped by technology of antenatal diagnosis.

A major epistemic novelty, brought about by the development of foetal diagnostics since the 1960s, is depiction of the *foetus* as a subject of life and health that is conceivable separately from the bodily processes and medical condition of the pregnant woman. The foetus in antenatal diagnosis and health care owes its existence to medical high-tech and is a profoundly epistemic and *technical* figure. It is regarded as a cluster of chromosomal, genetic, physiological and other 'factors' of life that only specific devices and techniques can make perceivable. Different medical specialities define the foetus on the molecular level as a kind of juncture of interaction between genetic information and chemical and physiological processes. The foetus is certainly conceived of as a living being but not as a person or individual (Mitchell 1994; Weir 1996). Rather, the figure of the foetus in contemporary reproductive medicine is a *dividual* (Deleuze 1995), an amalgamation of specific indications of basic, verifiable processes of life 'itself'. As such it functions as a point of reference that enables molecular findings and calculations of population and clinical risks to make sense in medical practice (see Kay 1993: 4–5; Rose 2001: 13).

When making a choice about foetal diagnosis the pregnant woman faces the figure of the foetus as *the other*. By making up the foetus through molecular findings and risk parameters, foetal diagnosis, as an agent of biomedical science, gives the uncertainty of life a form in which it is expressed as comprehensible and manageable. In a way, this form disguises the existential character of the woman's choice – its singularity and absoluteness – in a discursive matrix of rational choice. This rationale can be easily combined with the principles of informed consent and woman's choice. The affinity invokes the personal *responsibility* to calculate and manage objectively indicated risks in her own life.

However, the figure of the foetus that the pregnant woman faces refers to something beyond risk. To a remarkable extent, high-tech antenatal care fabricates the 'baby' that the pregnant woman can 'see' and experience as a distinct living being, as if real. This 'techno-foetus' stands for the other that is personally significant to her and tacitly felt by her. (For more detailed analysis, see Mitchell 1994; Mitchell and Georges 1998; Rapp 2000: 116–128; Helén 2004a: 40.) For this reason, the ethical problematization of the medical technology that essentially concerns the personal choice and the self cannot be restricted to risk-calculating responsibility. The latter is necessarily accompanied by existential responsibility that is characterized not by risk assessment but by *anxiety*.

Anxiety management

Anxiety in women's consent and choice is by no means a neglected aspect of foetal diagnosis but, on the contrary, a significant issue in contemporary obstetrical health care. When the use of foetal diagnostic techniques in gynaecological and obstetrical practice began to increase in the 1970s, a special discourse, counselling practice and expertise in dealing with the 'emotional side' of antenatal testing and screening emerged. The first studies on 'psychological sequelae' in women subjected to these procedures were conducted in the late 1970s and early 1980s, notably in the United States and Great Britain. Since the late 1980s, a special field of research in medical psychology has evolved concerning the use of ultrasound scan, amniocentesis, CVS, maternal serum blood test and DNA tests in maternity care and selective abortion. The range of topics of study is wide: adequacy of the information on screening and testing procedures that is given to patients; anxiety and stress in pregnant women during and after the procedure; attitudes towards pregnancy, the baby and the screening and testing procedures; 'factors' affecting the decisions of women to participate in the procedure and undergo abortion; and women's coping and capability to manage their own lives in cases of abortion or giving birth to a disabled child. Strikingly, these aspects of discussion and research were virtually non-existent in Finland until the late 1990s.[3]

These studies are textbook examples of a basic mechanism of psychologization (Rose 1996), since they give the cognitive or emotional phenomenon under study a measurable and calculable form by subjecting women to psychological tests. Numerous studies concentrate on the effects of antenatal screening and testing procedures on the emotions of the pregnant woman and on her attitudes towards pregnancy and the 'foetus' (in some studies, 'baby'). *Anxiety* emerges as a dominant theme, when women who are undergoing the procedure or who have received a 'false positive' result or who have been compelled to make a choice regarding 'selective' abortion are asked to describe their feelings during the process. Most of the studies used a psychological questionnaire test to rate women's 'anxiety level' and its changes during the procedure (the Spielberg State-Trait Anxiety Inventory has been the most popular). Similarily, many studies measure women's attitudes by a 'mother–foetal attachment scale'.

The basic finding is that antenatal screening and testing procedures cause pregnant women considerable anxiety. Should the test not indicate any foetal abnormality, anxiety is dispelled rapidly, implying that antenatal screening and testing could provide psychological 'reassurance' to the pregnant woman. However, in cases of selective abortion, the anxiety caused by the operation is far greater than in cases in which women have wanted abortion. In fact, the anxiety caused by selective abortion equals the 'anxiety level' of women who have given birth to a stillborn baby.

This discourse states, as a fact, that anxiety is involved in the procedure and is even an outcome of it. Hence, it makes anxiety material in high-tech reproductive medicine, but in such a manner that it seems to have hardly any connection to the ethical and existential dimension of choice. By regarding the anxiety engendered by women's situation in uncertainty and choice as an emotional reaction, this discourse *psychologizes* the choice. Further, anxiety is given a calculable form. The translation of anxiety into 'scales' and 'scores' makes it comprehensible in the practical context of reproductive medicine. It becomes a factor that is compatible with other factors involved and can be evaluated through risk calculation. Consequently, anxiety is transformed into a manageable and thus a technical matter.

Research on women's psychological reactions and psychosocial care to relieve the anxiety related to foetal diagnoses constitute a supplementary practice to hardcore biomedicine. Nevertheless, anxiety management is considered indispensable in facilitating the introduction of foetal diagnosis and antenatal screening techniques into routine operations of maternity care (see Petersen 1999). In Western medicine today, this mediation between technical novelties and routine practices is important in a particular sense. The rapid development of medical technology and emphasis on laboratory research and on the experimental aspects of medicine have opened up unforeseeable opportunities to engineer human bodies and life. This development has, in turn, created a threat that both the patient and the body will disappear from the horizon of contemporary biomedicine (see Williams 1997). Therefore, the task of supplementary practices like anxiety management is to bring bodies and patients back into the field of high-tech biomedicine, to hold patients and bodies still, so to speak. However, it also reinforces the tendency to view the problems in the implementation of high-tech medicine in such a manner that their locus is the life and existence of the individual person. It moreover suggests that these problems are manageable.

Ethics cum medical technology

The diverse manners by which significant issues of antenatal diagnosis and selective abortion are articulated as ethical problems reflect more generally the 'ethical' discussion in today's advanced biomedicine. Widespread adoption of informed consent and non-directiveness as the guiding principles of foetal diagnosis, genetic research and counselling, stem cell research and of collecting of samples and medical information for bio banks (e.g. Petersen 1999; Høyer 2003; Novas 2003: 89–107) is an indication of the need to make state-of-the-art medical technology morally acceptable. This preoccupation with ethics ensures that the potentially worrying or controversial aspects of medical high-tech do not obstruct the advance of biomedical science (Lemke 2000; Jallinoja 2002). In a sense, the articulation of problems and controversies in terms of ethics has overshadowed the political aspects.

In my study, however, I have drawn attention to other ethical aspects on high-tech medicine. The situation of choice, with the related anxiety, that a pregnant woman faces in the procedure of antenatal diagnosis and selective abortion is an example of ethical problems involved in medical technology that are connected with the personal existence of individuals, their lives, bodies and experiences. This ethical situation seems to be characteristic to high-tech reproductive medicine in general (Wrede 1997; Ruhl 1999), and to infertility treatment in particular (Franklin 1997). It is also comparable with many conditions that diagnostic testing based on molecular biology, ultrasound scanning, computer imagining and other advanced techniques enable to be detected and predicted before there is any notable or experienced symptoms of ill-health in the patient. The range of 'presymptomatic illness' (Nelkin 1993: 189) varies from HIV-positive to specific hereditary diseases like Huntington's chorea, and it is expanding greatly due to the notion of genetic illness (Yoxen 1984; Koch 1999; Lemke 2000: 236–238). Moreover, the way risk awareness is connected with personal choice in the procedure of antenatal diagnostic testing is an example of an existential condition that biomedical high-tech imposes also on the treatment of chronic diseases like diabetes and cancer (Mol 1998: 280–283).

A common element in all these conditions of high-tech health care is a mixture of prediction and promise that concerns personal life and health. Advanced biomedicine carries out predictive diagnosis to unveil a potential disease or a state of ill-health, conceived of as the health risk of an individual, irrespective of any symptoms. In a way, it has power to define the molecular destiny of the person. However, the medical machinery is also able to offer options to overcome and change this destiny, or offer support to cope with it. And an individual person has to make a choice about these options or, rather, promises.

Implicitly, these promises require from each individual person the anticipatory conduct of living. In other words, technics imposes an ethical practice that demands a person to live his or her own life beforehand (see Helén 2004a: 44–45; 2004b: 10–11) For such a 'care of the self' (Foucault 1997: 225–228), the idea of *risk* is indispensable, since it preserves uncertainty, included in many aspects of life and health, but tames it in a calculable and manageable form, thus making personal risk assessment possible. Furthermore, the implementation of advanced medical technology insinuates a tenet of *responsibilization*. This is well illustrated by the fact that antenatal diagnosis requires pregnant women to become individuals capable of transforming uncertainties of their lives into calculable options and of making choices (Beck-Gernsheim 1996: 289–290; Petersen 1998; Novas and Rose 2000: 502–507; see also O'Malley 1996).

However, in such an ethical practice the personal decisions required and the related anxiety are not defined only in terms of calculation or responsibility, guilt or sacrifice. In addition, the expectations concerning new medical knowledge of and cure for the person's disease-to-be are involved, with a perspective of hope and despair and with uncertainty that is not about life but about the moulding of life (Helén 2004b: 11, 17–18).

Hence, medical technology is imposed on matters concerning a person's relation to the self, to his or her own body, life and existence. Accordingly, significant problems in the field of high-tech medicine are defined in terms of personal existence. Furthermore, the only way to deal with these problems provided by our liberal rationale is through personal choice. This undoubtedly is a reason for the *ethical* perplexity and difficulty of pursuing the *politics* of high-tech biomedicine.

Notes

1 My research material consists of articles and other writings by Finnish physicians in Finnish and international medical journals on the subjects of antenatal screenings and diagnostic, as well as reviews by Finnish medical geneticists on developments in and prospects for their field. The guidelines for antenatal screening procedures set by public health authorities are also included. For a complete list of the texts included, see Helén (2002).

2 I refer particularly to the basic concepts of existentialist ethics as presented by Sartre (1956: 433–556, 625–628) and Beauvoir (1976) (see also Macquarrie, 1973: 177–188, 206–218).

3 For example, the list of references in Green and Statham (1996: 157–163) illustrates the range of this field of medical psychology. For a complete list of the texts on which my following excursus is based, see Helén (2002).

References

Asmala, K. (1995) "Downin oireyhtymän seulonta Suomessa", *Suomen Lääkärilehti*, 50(25): 2585–2588.

Aula, P. and Leisti, J. (1994) 'Mutaation tunnistamisesta väestön kartoitukseen', *Duodecim*, 110(7): 749–756.

Baker, T. and Simon, J. (2002) 'Embracing risk', in T. Baker and J. Simon (eds) *Embracing Risk: The Changing Culture of Insurance and Responsibility*. Chicago: University of Chicago Press.

Beauvoir, S. de (1976) *The Ethics of Ambiguity*. New York: Citadel.

Beck-Gernsheim, E. (1996) 'Die soziale Konstruktion des Risikos – das Beispiel Pränatal Diagnostik', *Soziale Welt*, 47(3): 284–296.

Chapelle, A. de la (1993) 'Disease gene mapping in isolated human populations: the example of Finland', *Journal of Medical Genetics*, 30(10): 857–865.

Cowan, R.S. (1993) 'Genetic technology and reproductive choice: an ethics of autonomy', in D. Kevles and L. Hood (eds) *The Code of Codes: Scientific and Social Issues in the Human Genome Project*. Cambridge, MA and London: Harvard University Press.

Deleuze, G. (1995) 'Postscript on control societies', in *Negotiations 1972–1990*. New York: Columbia University Press.

Dworkin, R. (2001) 'What is sacred?' in R. Harris (ed.) *Bioethics*. Oxford: Oxford University Press.

Eronen, H., Soimula, A. and Gissler, M. (2003) *Induced Abortions and Sterilisations 2002*. Statistical Summary 23/2003. Helsinki: National Research and Development Centre for Welfare and Health.

Ettorre, E. (1996) *New Genetics Discourse in Finland: Exploring Experts' Views within Surveillance Medicine*. Helsinki: Suomen Kuntaliitto.

Faden, R. (1991) 'Autonomy, choice, and the new reproductive technologies: the role of informed consent in prenatal genetic diagnosis', in J. Rodin and A. Collins (eds) *Women and New Reproductive Technologies: Medical, Psychosocial, Legal and Ethical Dilemmas*. Hillsdale, NJ: Lawrence Erlbaum.

Faden, R. and Beauchamp, T. (1986) *A History and Theory of Informed Consent*. New York: Oxford University Press.

Flower, M.J. and Heath, D. (1993) 'Micro-anatomo politics: mapping of the Human Genome Project', *Culture, Medicine and Psychiatry*, 17(1): 27–41.

Franklin, S. (1997) *Embodied Progress: A Cultural Account of Assisted Conception*. London and New York: Routledge.

Foucault, M. (1985) *The Use of Pleasure*. New York: Pantheon.

Foucault, M. (1997) 'Technologies of the self', in *Ethics: Essential Works of Michel Foucault 1*. London: Allen Lane.

Garland, D. (2003) 'The rise of risk', in R.V. Ericsson and A. Doyle (eds) *Risk and Morality*. Toronto: Toronto University Press.

Gissler, M., Toukomaa, H. and Virtanen, M. (1996) *Finnish Perinatal Statistics 1995*. Helsinki: STAKES.

Green, J. and Statham, H. (1996) 'Psychosocial aspects of prenatal screening and diagnosis', in T. Marteau and M. Richards (eds) *The Troubled Helix: Social and Psychological Implications of the New Human Genetics*. Cambridge: Cambridge University Press.

Helén, I. (2002) 'Risk and anxiety: polyvalence of ethics in high-tech antenatal care', *Critical Public Health*, 12(2): 119–137.

Helén, I. (2004a) 'Technics over life: risk, ethics and the existential condition in high-tech antenatal care', *Economy and Society*, 33(1): 28–51.

Helén, I. (2004b) 'Health in prospect: high-tech medicine, life enhancement and the economy of hope', *Science Studies*, 17(1): 3–19.

Helén, I. and Yesilova, K. (2003) 'Vietti, väestö ja valinta: seksuaaliterveyden kerrostumat Suomessa', in I. Helén and M. Jauho (eds) *Kansalaisuus ja kansanterveys*. Helsinki: Gaudeamus.

Hemminki, E., Malin, M. and Kojo-Austin, H. (1990) 'Prenatal care in Finland: from primary to tertiary health care', *International Journal of Health Services*, 20(2): 221–232.

Høyer, K. (2003) '"Science is really needed, that's all I know": informed consent and non-verbal practices of collecting blood samples for genetic research in Northern Sweden', *New Genetics and Society*, 22(3): 229–244.

Hubbard, R. (1990) *The Politics of Women's Biology*. New Brunswick, NJ: Rutgers University Press.

Jallinoja, P. (2001) 'Genetic screening in maternity care: preventive aims and voluntary choices', *Sociology of Health and Illness*, 23(3): 286–307.

Jallinoja, P. (2002) 'Ethics of clinical genetics and genetic research: the spirit of profession and trials of suitability from 1970 to 2000', *Critical Public Health*, 12(2): 103–118.

Kay, L. (1993) *The Molecular Vision of Life*. New York and Oxford: Oxford University Press.

Kevles, D. (1993) 'Out of eugenics: the historical politics of the human genome', in D. Kevles and L. Hood (eds) *The Code of Codes: Scientific and Social Issues in the Human Genome Project*. Cambridge, MA and London: Harvard University Press.

Koch, L. (1999) 'Predictive genetic medicine: a new concept of disease', in E. Hildt and S. Graumann (eds) *Genetics in Human Reproduction*. Aldershot: Ashgate.

Koch, L. and Stemerding, D. (1994) 'The sociology of entrenchment: a cystic fibrosis test for everyone?' *Social Science & Medicine*, 39(9): 1211–1220.

Lemke, T. (2000) 'Die Regierung der Risiken: von der Eugenik zur genetischen Gouvernementalität', in U. Bröckling, S. Krasmann and T. Lemke (eds) *Gouvernementalität der Gegenwart: Studien zur Ökonomisierung des Sozialen*. Frankfurt am Main: Suhrkamp.

Lippman, A. (1991) 'Prenatal testing and screening: constructing needs and reinforcing inequities', *American Journal of Law and Medicine*, 17(1): 15–50.

Luker, K. (1985) *Abortion and Politics of Motherhood*. Berkeley, CA: University of California Press.

Macquarrie, J. (1973) *Existentialism*. London: Penguin.

Ministry of Social Affairs and Health (1998) *Geeniseulontatyöryhmän muistio* (Workgroup of genetic screening: a memo). Helsinki: Ministry of Social Affairs and Health.

Mitchell, L.M. (1994) 'The routinitization of the other: ultrasound, women and the fetus', in G. Basen, M. Eichler and A. Lippman (eds) *Misconceptions: The Social Construction of Choice and the New Reproductive and Genetic Technologies*, vol. 2. Prescott, ON: Voyageur.

Mitchell, L.M., and Georges, E. (1998) 'Baby's first picture: the cyborg fetus of ultrasound imaging', in R. Davis-Floyd and J. Dumit (eds) *Cyborg-Babies: From Techno-Sex to Techno-Tots*. New York and London: Routledge.

Mol, A. (1998) 'Lived reality and the multiplicity of norms: a critical tribute to Georges Canguilhem', *Economy and Society*, 27(2–3): 274–284.

Nelkin, D. (1993) 'The social power of genetic information', in D. Kevles and L. Hood (eds) *The Code of Codes: Scientific and Social Issues in the Human Genome Project*. Cambridge, MA and London: Harvard University Press.

Novas, C. (2003) 'Governing "risky" genes: predictive genetics, counselling expertise and the care of the self', PhD thesis, Department of Sociology, Goldsmiths College, University of London.

Novas, C. and Rose, N. (2000) 'Genetic risk and the birth of the somatic individual', *Economy and Society*, 29(4): 485–513.

Oakley, A. (1993) *Essays on Women, Medicine and Health*. Edinburgh: Edinburgh University Press.

O'Malley, P. (1996) 'Risk and responsibility', in A. Barry, T. Osborne and N. Rose (eds) *Foucault and Political Reason: Liberalism, Neo-liberalisn and Rationalities of Government*. London: UCL Press.

Overall, C. (1987) *Ethics and Human Reproduction: A Feminist Analysis*. London: Allen & Unwin.

Petersen, A. (1998) 'The new genetics and the politics of public health', *Critical Public Health*, 8(1): 59–71.

Petersen, A. (1999) 'Counselling genetically "at-risk": the poetics and politics of "non-directiveness"', *Health, Risk & Society*, 1(3): 253–266.

Rabinow, P. (1996) 'Artificiality and enlightenment: from sociobiology to biosociality', in *Essays on the Anthropology of Reason*. Princeton, NJ: Princeton University Press.

Rapp, R. (2000) *Testing Women, Testing the Fetus: The Social Impact of Amniocentesis in America*. New York and London: Routledge.

Rheinberger, H-J. (1995) 'Beyond nature and culture: a note on medicine in the age of molecular biology', *Science in Context*, 8(1): 249–263.

Rose, N. (1996) *Inventing our Selves: Psychology, Power, and Personhood*. Cambridge and New York: Cambridge University Press.

Rose, N. (2001) 'The politics of life itself', *Theory, Culture & Society*, 18(6): 1–30.

Rothman, B.K. (1996) *The Tentative Pregnancy: Amniocentesis and the Sexual Politics of Motherhood*. London: Pandora and HarperCollins.

Ruhl, L. (1999) 'Liberal governance and prenatal care: risk and regulation of pregnancy', *Economy and Society*, 28(1): 95–117.

Santalahti, P. and Hemminki. E. (1998) 'Use of prenatal screening tests in Finland', *European Journal of Public Health*, 8(1): 8–14.

Sartre, J-P. (1956) *Being and Nothingness*. New York: Philosophical Library.

STAKES (1995) *Seulontatutkimukset ja yhteistyö äitiyshuollossa*. Helsinki: National Research and Development Centre for Welfare and Health.

STAKES (1996) *Reproduction and its Trends: Statistics on Pregnancies, Childbirths, Sterilisations and Congenital Malformations in Finland*. Helsinki: National Research and Development Centre for Welfare and Health.

STAKES (1999) *Seulontatutkimukset ja yhteistyö äitiyshuollossa*. Helsinki: National Research and Development Centre for Welfare and Health.

Syvänen, A-C., Ikonen, E., Manninen, T., Bengström, M., Söderlund, H., Aula, P. and Peltonen, L. (1992) 'Convenient and quantitative determination of the frequency of a mutant allele using solid-phase minisequencing: application to aspartylglucosaminuria in Finland, *Genomics*, 12(3): 590–595.

Weir, L. (1996) 'Recent developments in the government of pregnancy', *Economy and Society*, 25(3): 372–392.

Williams, S.J. (1997) 'Modern medicine and the "uncertain body": from corporeality to hyperreality?', *Social Science & Medicine*, 45(7): 1041–1049.

Wrede, S. (1997) 'The notion of risk in Finnish prenatal care: managing risk mothers and risk pregnancies', in E. Riska (ed.) *Images of Women's Health: The Social Construction of Gendered Health*. Åbo: Institute of Women's Studies at Åbo Akademi.

Yoxen, E.J. (1984) 'Constructing genetic diseases', in T. Duster and K. Garrett (eds) *Cultural Perspectives on Biological Knowledge*. Norwood, NJ: Ablex.

Chapter 3

The first genetic screening in Finland

Its execution, evaluation and some possible implications for liberal government

Seppo Poutanen

Introduction

Genetic screening is no novelty to the world. In the medical literature, the following cases are often produced as examples of success in the field:

- *Beta-thalassemia:* carrier frequency of this inherited haemoglobin disorder is high in some Mediterranean populations. In Sardinia, in 1977, for example, voluntary screening was made available to young unmarried adults, prospective parents and couples with an ongoing pregnancy (Hietala 1998).
- *Cystic fibrosis (CF):* the gene behind this chronic lung disease and pancreatic insufficiency was cloned in 1989. During the 1990s, several pilot CF studies were performed in many countries (Hietala 1998).

None of the diseases mentioned, or their screening, has much relevance to native Finns, because the properties of the Finnish gene pool are in many respects different from the genetic features of other populations (Norio et al. 1973). This chapter first describes how some Finnish geneticists planned and executed the first pilot genetic screening in Finland. Concerning my efforts to then analyse some possible implications of their work, it must be noted that by the first years of the twenty-first century, practices of genetic screening had been established on only a small scale in Finland (Jallinoja 2002). The reasons for this relative standstill deserve studies of their own.

The geneticists and some Finnish social scientists agree that the general public should get more information on the nature of genetics. This recommendation is, however, problematic, because genetic information is very complex. Applying standard bioethics I argue that if a person is offered genetic screening, she should get a chance to consider the information with some helpful method. I then introduce so-called Bayesian decision analysis as such a potential method and demonstrate its use (as far as I know, the analysis is not actually practised in this way anywhere – not yet, at least).

Finally, this chapter interprets the problem of distributing and understanding genetic information in the context of *(neo)liberal government* (e.g. Rose 1998; Dean 1999). Raising people's consciousness of genes, and providing them with the means to manage their genetic risks by launching genetic screening, can be seen to manifest this type of government. Furthermore, I hold the idea of offering Bayesian decision analysis to people who ponder participation in genetic screening to fit well with liberal government, because the point of Bayesian decision analysis is to help people to become more autonomous, i.e. *self-governing*. I do not, however, evaluate genetic screening, Bayesian decision analysis or liberal government ethically or politically, but I outline one possible development in genetic health care.

Launching the AGU pilot screening in Finland

Visions of Finnish geneticists

In 1994, Pertti Aula, Professor of Medical Genetics, and Jaakko Leisti, Docent of Genetics, outlined the future of genetic screening in Finland. According to them, the goal of such screening is to diminish the emergence of hereditary diseases among the population, but this goal cannot be reached without building a suitable infrastructure. Aula and Leisti (1994) state that, first, this process should begin by raising Finns' awareness of hereditary diseases and the possibilities of genetics. In an ideal situation, the national school system would inform young people, so that they would be able to understand any future screening programme correctly. Second, there must be facilities for informing and counselling individuals who participate in screening, and also resources for diagnosing pregnancies. Third, an organization and diagnostic laboratories are needed for collecting and transporting genetic samples (Aula and Leisti 1994).

In the geneticists' opinion, to include genetic screening in state-funded health services would be the best way to guarantee an equal chance of participation for all concerned. Consequently, Aula and Leisti complain about the lack of a general physical examination, which would cover all young adults before they start planning a family. It would be relatively easy to screen almost all young men, because there is obligatory military service in Finland, but the geneticists do not regard screening of conscripts as a serious option. This is because they see young women to be mainly responsible for family planning. Additionally, they consider there to be ethical and practical reasons against including genetic screening in the school health service and so, ultimately, the only justifiable and practically feasible site for screening is the maternity clinic (Aula and Leisti 1994). Aula and Leisti summarize their recommendations as follows:

> An organization of foetal diagnostics has already operated with great success for almost twenty years in Finland, and it has created a good infrastructure

> for co-operation between prenatal care, clinical genetics and chromosome laboratories. It is most desirable that possible genetic screening also be carried out in the setting of maternity clinics and the public health service.
>
> (Aula and Leisti 1994: 754, translation SP)

The geneticists also focus on different ethical dimensions of genetic screening, and they stress the need for it to be voluntary, with respect for participants' autonomy and measures against discrimination. In conclusion, Aula and Leisti predict the future of genetic screening to be quite linear in Finland: limits to the introduction of screening will be set only by the rate of technological development and economic resources (Aula and Leisti 1994).

Goals of the AGU screening and opinions of the Finnish public about genetic screening

The planning of the first genetic screening in Finland was already under way when Aula and Leisti wrote their article. This pilot screening was launched during 1994–1995, and according to Marja Hietala, a geneticist centrally responsible for performing the study, the aims of the project were:

> To evaluate the carrier frequency of aspartylglucosaminuria (AGU) in Finland and to detect potential regional differences . . . to explore attitudes toward genetic testing among the general population and relatives of AGU patients . . . to evaluate the attitudes and experiences of the women to whom the gene test was offered . . . to evaluate the feasibility of a genetic screening program in primary health care using AGU carrier screening of pregnant women as the model.
>
> (Hietala 1998: 39)

AGU is, according to Hietala, 'a severe disorder leading to progressive mental retardation and . . . to institutional care in adult age . . . only symptomatic treatment is available at the moment' (Hietala 1998: 38). AGU is inherited recessively, which means that a person will get the disease only in the case that she/he inherits a mutated DNA sequence from both of her/his parents. If a man and a woman are both carriers of this gene defect, then there is a 25 per cent probability that their child will get AGU (Ikonen and Palotie 1994). There are several hereditary diseases over-represented in the Finnish gene pool and usually only one major genetic mutation behind these diseases. Therefore, geneticists consider this pool to offer excellent opportunities for screening, and AGU is a representative example of Finnish gene defects (Hietala et al. 1995, 1996; Hietala 1998).

The general questionnaire study in the project asked these main questions: (1) to whom and when genetic tests should be offered, (2) reasons for or against gene testing and (3) concerns about genetic testing (Hietala et al. 1995). In what follows, I will briefly summarize some of the results in respect to every question:

- *Question 1:* about 90 per cent of all respondents agreed with the statement 'gene testing should be available to anybody who wishes to have information about the disease genes she/he carries'. However, 17 per cent of the population, but only 4 per cent of the relatives of patients with AGU, accepted the view that 'gene tests should not be performed at all' (Hietala et al. 1995).
- *Question 2:* primarily, the respondents wanted to influence their own or their offspring's health and life, but 60 per cent of all were also willing to use gene tests to save society health care costs. The main reasons expressed against testing were the danger of discrimination in employment or in insurance policies, and a possible increase in selective abortions (Hietala et al. 1995).
- *Question 3:* the respondents' biggest concern about gene testing was caused by the possibility of 'eugenics': 80 per cent overall were somewhat or very worried about this. (For some reason, the researchers did not give any definition of 'eugenics'.) Furthermore, people were also somewhat worried about the possibility of genetic information ending up in the wrong hands (Hietala et al. 1995).

In their final discussion, the researchers conclude, 'the present questionnaire survey indicated that the Finnish population . . . have a positive attitude toward genetic testing in risk determination for a variety of genetically determined disorders' (Hietala et al. 1995: 1497). Hietala et al. suggest this approval derives from the overall positive attitude of Finns towards the national health care system, which provides equalized opportunities for high-quality public health care.

Experiences of mothers and recommendations for the future

The pilot carrier screening for the AGU gene mutation was performed at two maternity health care centres in Helsinki, the capital of Finland. Before the screening, the personnel of maternity care units and health centre laboratories were given some information on gene testing and the AGU disease. The gene test, which requires taking a blood sample from a finger, was offered to 2077 native Finnish women during early pregnancy, 1975 (95 per cent) of whom chose to participate. As a result, 31 carriers of the AGU gene mutation were detected, but partners of the carrier women, who consequently agreed to be tested, were found not to be carriers (Hietala 1998; Hietala et al. 1998).

Most women who answered a questionnaire study found the decision on whether to participate or not 'easy' or 'rather easy' (92 per cent of the participants, 79 per cent of the decliners). The most crucial reasons for the women to participate were a need to ensure that the baby would be healthy, and a willingness to participate in every test offered by maternity care. On the other hand, the women who refused the test were mainly worried about a possible decision to terminate the pregnancy (Hietala 1998; Hietala et al. 1998). Concerning background variables, Hietala notes that 'there were no significant differences in socio-demographic variables between participants and decliners' (Hietala 1998: 55).

Although the decliners expressed more critical attitudes on genetic testing (e.g. pointing to unnecessary anxieties), the women in both groups agreed that pregnancy was not the best time for such a thing. Instead, they considered the family planning period more optimal (Hietala et al. 1998). Hietala states that several disorders in the Finnish disease heritage might reasonably be included in genetic screening with AGU. According to her, the proper performance of future screening will require giving adequate information to possible participants in all relevant contexts, and careful consideration of the purpose and the psychosocial and ethical aspects of each programme by performing professionals (Hietala 1998).

How an argument for offering Bayesian decision analysis to intended subjects of genetic screening can be derived from medical and social scientists' views

Recommendation to distribute more genetic and related information

The point of departure for my analysis in the rest of this chapter is the premise that there prevails a certain agreement among the geneticists and some of those Finnish social scientists who have studied genetics-related phenomena. The agreement is expressed not only by Aula and Leisti (1994) and Hietala (1998), but also by Jallinoja et al. (1998) and Jallinoja and Aro (2000) as a recommendation of this kind: the general public/school pupils/pregnant women/nurses in maternity care/other performing professionals should get more factual/ethical/other kinds of information on the nature of genetics/genetic screening. The recommendation may seem unproblematic and ethically sound, but I show how more genetic information is prone to intensify the puzzling nature of some situations involving choice. I assume it to follow from standard bioethics that people who face such difficult choices should be helped, and I introduce Bayesian decision analysis as an aid that seems appropriate.

First, Aula and Leisti base the recommendation both on their goal of fighting hereditary diseases and on the recommendations of CAHBI (1991: CAHBI is the ad hoc Committee of Experts on Bioethics under the Council of Europe), which stress the voluntary nature of screening and respect for participants' autonomy. Second, Hietala agrees with the stated moral principles, but in addition she and her research team can refer to their questionnaire studies. For instance, regarding knowledge gaps, five of the twenty-five women who were found to be carriers of the AGU gene mutation and who responded to the questionnaire thought that they had not got enough information before the test (Hietala et al. 1998).

In the social scientific research, a central subject of discussion has been the attitudes of Finns towards genetic testing. Jallinoja et al. (1998) found contradictory attitudes, sometimes taken by the same individuals, and a recommendation is therefore given that 'it is important that health professionals . . . help their clients cope with contradictory feelings and help them find an acceptable solution for their specific life situation' (Jallinoja et al. 1998: 1372). In another study, Jallinoja and Aro (2000) examined Finns' comprehension of basic genetics. The researchers then analysed the relationship between levels of knowledge and attitudes towards gene tests. In their conclusions, they recommend that, in addition to improving everybody's ability to seek and understand genetic knowledge, citizens should also be provided with 'tools to perceive and discuss potential ethical and social problems, which . . . genetic testing and screening bring along' (Jallinoja and Aro 2000: 29).

Possibilities to improve the information distributed to subjects of the AGU screening

Mothers who were the intended subjects of the AGU pilot screening were told about the matter during their first visit to a maternity care unit, or they got an information leaflet by post afterwards (Hietala et al. 1996). The leaflet discloses these facts, for example:

- 2 per cent (1 in 50) of Finns carry the AGU gene defect
- only about 200 people have ever been found to suffer from the AGU disease in Finland
- if both a child's parents carry the gene defect, then she/he has a one in four risk of inheriting the defect from both her/his parents and thus becoming ill with the AGU disease
- there is a test that can find the gene mutation in healthy carriers
- the AGU disease can be detected prenatally from a foetus by examining the placenta or amniotic fluid (Hietala 1998).

Accordingly, the leaflet gave *probabilities* that range from quite large (one in four) to obviously rather small (in the light of the given facts, the probability of having a child with the AGU disease is approximately $1/50 \times 1/50 \times 1/4 = 1/10{,}000$ for most native Finns), but the women were presented with apparent *certainties*, too: a test will find the gene mutation, and there are methods to decide whether a foetus has got the disease. As regards these probabilities, their interpretation is clearly no straightforward matter, but if the leaflet had been more detailed, that is, if the women had received more information, the facts that needed grasping would essentially have become more complicated.

To start with the first fact in the leaflet, different studies have actually given different values to the carrier frequency of the AGU gene mutation among Finns, the range having varied from 1/30 to 1/70 (Syvänen et al. 1992; Hietala et al. 1995; Hietala 1998). Because regional differences have also been found (Hietala 1998), an individual who would like to know the probability of her/his carrying the AGU gene mutation as precisely as possible should study the history of her/his family and look for relatives who might have had the AGU disease.

The distinction between probabilities and certainties posited in the leaflet breaks down because detection of the AGU gene mutation cannot be *absolutely* reliable, a fact that has nothing special to do with the AGU gene test but concerns all diagnostic medical tests. The reliability of such tests is measured in two dimensions called 'sensitivity' and 'specificity',[1] and these cannot be protected perfectly against the possibility of errors. One distinguishing source of mistakes is in fact built into the AGU gene test, for the gene mutation that the test detects is not responsible for *all* AGU diseases in the Finnish population. Instead, 1 per cent of the Finnish AGU cases are caused by undetectable gene mutations (Isoniemi et al. 1995; Hietala et al. 1996; Valkonen et al. 1999). This means, using established terminology, that the sensitivity of a technically faultless AGU gene test is 99 per cent.

The aforesaid also holds true for detecting the AGU disease in a foetus, but an additional piece of information deserves attention. Namely, that to get samples directly from foetal tissue is not harmless, and there exists a risk of miscarriage. In Finland it has been estimated that the probability of miscarriage caused by taking a sample from a placenta or amniotic fluid is 1 per cent on average (Teikari 2003). When it comes to individual cases, this may mean that a mother pondering over the health of her foetus learns that her risk of miscarriage may be significantly higher than 1 per cent.

How Bayesian decision analysis deals with implied problems

The more detailed information on the AGU and its testing a person gets, the more complicated her/his choice situation will apparently become. This state of affairs can be taken as grounds (in line with Jallinoja and Aro's recommendations, for instance) for equipping potential testees with 'tools' for understanding the facts, and the individual, social, ethical, etc. consequences of alternative choices. What might such tools be like? Should these potential testees be taught different ethical theories, for example? But would it be justifiable to confront, for example, a strongly religious person with claims of secular ethics? On the other hand, at least one requirement derives from standard bioethical recommendations of respect for a person's freedom and autonomy: an acceptable tool must not *in itself* favour any alternative at the expense of others.

One optional tool that fulfils the stated requirement is a certain decision-making method, which is sometimes called Bayesian decision analysis (e.g. Bell et al. 1988). The method is now applicable, because the choice of a person who considers participation in the AGU gene test is *uncertain*: without participating she/he will not know about some possible health risks of her/his offspring, but no test can give absolutely definitive results. According to the analysis, the basic steps to follow in this kind of uncertain situation are, first, determine probabilities 0–1 for all possible outcomes of different choices, second, evaluate the utility or disutility of the possible outcomes quantitatively, and third, determine the expected utility or disutility of every possible outcome through multiplying the quantified values of the outcomes by the probabilities of those outcomes. The rational decision is to make a choice from which the biggest combined utility or the smallest combined disutility will be expected (e.g. Bell et al. 1988).

For example, a pregnant woman who considers participation in the AGU screening could use the analysis in the following simple way. To begin with, the person – I will call her Mari – realizes that the risk of her having a baby with the AGU disease is constituted by three probabilities: her own probability of carrying the AGU gene mutation (1/50), her partner's probability of carrying the AGU gene mutation (1/50) and a baby's probability of getting the AGU disease if both its parents carry the AGU gene mutation (1/4). Accordingly, Mari's risk of having a baby with the AGU disease is approximately $1/50 \times 1/50 \times 1/4 = 1/10,000$.

Is the probability of 1/10,000 large or small? Mari does not need to answer this question, because the method processes probabilities as such. Instead, she must give numeric values to all possible outcomes of the choices available to her.[2] First, Mari can choose to participate in the AGU screening, or not to do so. In the simplified case here, she decides that possible outcomes of participating in the screening are having a baby without the AGU disease and getting a foetus with the AGU disease aborted. Respectively, the possible outcomes of not participating are having a baby without the AGU disease and having a baby with the AGU disease.

Let us suppose that Mari evaluates the birth of a baby with the AGU disease to be the worst possible outcome and describes the disutility of this happening with the number 100. On the other hand, because she sees no disutility in having a baby without the disease, it is logical to give number 0 to this possible outcome. To Mari's mind, getting an abortion is an unwanted result for any kind of reason, but not as bad a thing as having a baby with the AGU disease. Therefore, she decides to give a disutility of 70 to getting a foetus with the AGU disease aborted.

Mari can now count the expected disutilities of the choices open to her. First, the expected disutility of participating in the AGU screening is (70 × 1/10,000) + (0 × 9,999/10,000) = 0.007. And second, the expected disutility of not participating in the AGU screening is (100 × 1/10,000) + (0 × 9,999) = 0.01. To conclude, because the preceding expected disutility is smaller than the latter one, it is rational for Mari to participate in the AGU screening.

If applied in a way more sensitive to complications, the analysis could, for instance, make good use of the estimated sensitivity and specificity of the AGU gene test, and thus give Mari a chance to evaluate the reliability of her (or her partner's or foetus's) gene test results in advance as part of decision-making. Besides, she would not need to fix only one value on any of the relevant probabilities or on utilities/disutilities connected to the possible outcomes of the choices available to her. A sensible way to proceed might be to decide on as realistic and acceptable *ranges* of values as possible for different variables, and then to examine how moving between the extreme values will change the recommendation given by the analysis regarding rational choice.

Towards understanding Finnish genetic screening in the context of liberal government

Shortcomings in information distribution as a problem of liberal government

What sense – beyond appealing to some supposedly correct and shared bioethics – could be made of the Finnish geneticists' and social scientists' recommendation to distribute genetic and related information to virtually all Finns? How should the suggested role of Bayesian decision analysis be understood? One interesting and relevant viewpoint has been called *an analytics of liberal government* (e.g. Rose 1998; Dean 1999). According to Dean, 'analytics' now equals 'an analysis of the specific conditions under which particular entities emerge, exist and change' (Dean 1999: 20), and 'liberal government' means, to put it most simply, 'governing *through* the freedom and aspirations of subjects rather than in spite of them' (Rose 1998: 155).[3]

Consequently, the medical and social scientific studies I have described can be seen to indicate some emerging and potential ways of producing and governing Finns as free and autonomous, that is, self-governing subjects in their various relationships with a rapidly growing knowledge of the Finnish gene pool. From this viewpoint, the researchers' recommendation for information distribution is a way of contributing at a basic level to the production and government of Finns as such subjects. A person's freedom and autonomy are now thought to be manifested in her/his *personal choices*, but choices can be a person's own only if they are based on relevant and sufficient information.

The production of apt citizens does not, of course, need to start from scratch, because Finns already govern themselves in a mainly liberal way in their contacts with non-genetic medicine. Accordingly, as we have seen, Aula and Leisti (1994) can express their satisfaction with the fact that 'an organization of foetal diagnostics has already operated with great success for almost twenty years in Finland, and it has created a good infrastructure for co-operation between prenatal care, clinical genetics and chromosome laboratories' (Aula and Leisti 1994: 754) for a good reason. A complex assemblage of different medical techniques, various medical professionals with their consultative and treating expertise, administrative arrangements, physical spaces, etc. has already established what pregnancy is 'really' about in its ontological, epistemic and practical dimensions. This assemblage has also aimed to govern pregnant women as free and autonomous subjects who must make up their own minds in relation to 'conventional' prenatal tests.

The empirical studies described show Finns' knowledge of genetics to be relatively good, even if the general population had not yet been subjected to any genetic screening. From the liberal governmental viewpoint, however, shortcomings were also revealed. For instance, part of Jallinoja and Aro's (2000) results can be understood to mean that a significant number of Finns barely existed yet as liberally qualified subjects in relation to the emerging genetic dimension of their lives (compare e.g. Novas and Rose 2000).

When it comes to the AGU pilot screening, there is clearly something wrong with the two most important grounds for the mothers' participation in a way that intensifies the problem of governing them as free and autonomous individuals. First, the 'objective' function of the AGU screening is not to ensure the health of children, but to detect the AGU gene mutation, and second, a woman who wants to accept *any* test offered by maternity care will allow many choices to be made on her behalf. The intensification of the problem of liberal government now means that, on the one hand, distributing more information on the AGU gene mutation and the gene test would obviously not be enough to make women's decision-making 'right', but, on the other hand, if women were advised to 'correct' their thinking, this would violate the upheld liberal ideal of so-called non-directiveness in medical counselling.

Solution or further problems?

The main reason why I illustrated Bayesian decision analysis is that the method now reveals itself as *a potential liberal governmental technique* to apply to the problem outlined. A practical beginning to this would be to offer the method for mothers' use at maternity clinics, a move that could be justified – in line with standard bioethics – in two ways at least:

- To give quantitative utilities/disutilities to all possible outcomes of one's choices obviously requires imagining these outcomes as if they were

real, and so a mother who uses decision analysis will find it difficult to keep the illusion that screening simply secures a healthy child.
- To offer the method for mothers' use would not in itself direct their decision-making in any substantial sense. On the contrary, it has been argued that 'decision analysis can help reduce the influence of physicians on patient's decisions, by providing a quasi-independent source of advice' (Ubel and Loewenstein 1997: 650).

A pregnant woman who tried decision analysis and found its conceptualization of her situation appropriate and useful would be a 'success story' for not exactly liberal, but rather *neoliberal* government. Distinctions made between the two forms of government are rather vague in the literature, but the latter is associated with the following features at least: stress on individual choice, personal responsibility and control over one's own fate, extension of 'market rationality' to all spheres of life, and understanding life as a project of security against risks (e.g. Gordon 1991; O'Malley 1996; Petersen 1997).

But the question now arises, of course, as to whether there are or will be significant empirical preconditions for realization of such 'success stories'. Would any (Finnish) woman like to deal with her pregnancy by means of Bayesian decision analysis? If an expert tried to make sense of the method to a layperson, would this not actually mean directing the person and thus simultaneously violating the ideal of non-directiveness in medical counselling? Could (neo)liberal government ever become so perfect a regime (in Finland) that people would understand childbearing as a sphere of 'market rationality', in which consumer choices are made with the help of mathematical methods? Analysing many significant problems is beyond this chapter, but one point might be stressed. Namely, if the analysts of liberal government are right in their insistence on the strong historicality of subjects, identities, etc., then there can be neither 'natural' nor 'metaphysical' obstacles to hinder people from becoming fully trained Bayesians in any sphere of life.

Conclusion

From describing the visions of the planners of pilot genetic screening in Finland and the execution of it, I have come to understand genetic screening as an emerging form of liberal government. According to my interpretation, the essential problem from the point of view of liberal government here concerns information or knowledge: how the complicated facts about genetics and genetic screening and tests should be delivered to laypersons and how they could be made to understand and use these facts 'correctly'. My suggestion that liberal government could reasonably find Bayesian decision analysis to be part of the solution is speculative, but I have tried to demonstrate certain rationality based on standard bioethics that might lead to giving the subjects of genetic screening a chance to use the analysis.

Acknowledgements

I would like to thank Elizabeth Ettorre, Piia Jallinoja, Anne Kovalainen and Malcolm Williams for fruitful discussions, Alan Petersen for useful comments, and Academy of Finland for funding.

Notes

1 Let us suppose that there are 100 cases of a gene mutation and that a test is able to detect 99 of these cases. The test sensitivity is thus 0.99, which is the probability that a person gets a positive test result if she/he really has the gene mutation. In another group, we have 100 cases of a normal gene, and the test can show that 98 of these cases are normal. We have now the specificity of the test, i.e. 0.98, which is the probability that a person will get a negative test result, if she/he really has the normal gene (e.g. Bell et al. 1988).

2 There is no doubt that to evaluate 'quantitatively' such a possible outcome of one's choices as, for instance, giving birth to a disabled child would be difficult or impossible to many people. To begin with, what would be the units for counting? In my view, the role of numbers might be that of describing or symbolizing relative 'weights' in some intuitively acceptable manner. For example, most people would supposedly find it relatively easy to put these three illnesses in order regarding their 'disutility': a short bout of 'flu, asthma and leukaemia. In addition, however, many would probably like to say that leukaemia causes a lot more harm than the other two. Indicated 'distances' between the illnesses might then be put in proportion with each other on a numeric scale, e.g. 1 for 'flu, 4 for asthma and 10 for leukaemia on the 'disutility' scale of 0–10. For some suggested techniques to estimate different utilities/disutilities see e.g. Naglie et al. (1997).

3 In this analytic framework, such related entities as 'individuality', 'subjectivity', 'self', 'identity', 'autonomy' and 'freedom', for example, are taken to be empirical and historical phenomena (e.g. Foucault 1991; Fox 1997). Dean clarifies the meaning of 'governing subjects through their freedom' in this way:

> A useful way of thinking about liberalism as a regime of government ... is to consider the multiple ways it works through and attempts to construct a world of autonomous individuals, of 'free subjects'. This is a subject whose freedom is a condition of subjection. The exercise of authority presupposes the existence of a free subject of need, desire, rights, interests and choice. However, its subjection is also a condition of freedom: in order to act freely, the subject must first be shaped, guided and moulded into one capable of responsibly exercising that freedom through systems of domination. Subjection and subjectification are laid upon one another.
>
> (Dean 1999: 164–165).

It should also be noted that liberal government is, among other things, one general framework, in which so-called biopolitical goals are set and pursued (e.g. Foucault 1980; Turner 1997; Rose 2001).

References

Aula, P. and Leisti, J. (1994) 'Mutaation tunnistamisesta väestön kartoitukseen', *Duodecim*, 110: 749–756.

Bell, D.E., Raiffa, H. and Tversky, A. (1988) *Decision Making: Descriptive, Normative and Prescriptive Interactions*. Cambridge and New York: Cambridge University Press.

CAHBI (1991) *Recommendation No. R92(3)*. Brussels: Council of Europe.

Dean, M. (1999) *Governmentality: Power and Rule in Modern Society*. London and Thousand Oaks, CA: Sage.

Foucault, M. (1980) *The History of Sexuality, Volume One: An Introduction*, trans. R. Hurley. New York: Vintage.

Foucault, M. (1991) 'Governmentality', trans. R. Braidotti, in G. Burchell, C. Gordon and P. Miller (eds.) *The Foucault Effect: Studies in Governmentality*. Chicago, IL: University of Chicago Press.

Fox, N.J. (1997) 'Is there life after Foucault? Texts, frames and differends', in A. Petersen and R. Bunton (eds.) *Foucault, Health and Medicine*. London and New York: Routledge.

Gordon, C. (1991) 'Governmental rationality: an introduction', in G. Burchell, C. Gordon and P. Miller (eds.) *The Foucault Effect: Studies in Governmentality*. Chicago, IL: University of Chicago Press.

Hietala, M. (1998) *Prospects for Genetic Screening in Finland: Evaluation of the Feasibility of Carrier Screening in Primary Health Care using Aspartylglucosaminuria as the Model*. Turku: University of Turku.

Hietala, M., Hakonen, A., Aro, A.R., Niemelä, P., Peltonen, L. and Aula, P. (1995) 'Attitudes toward genetic testing among the general population and relatives of patients with a severe genetic disease: a survey from Finland', *American Journal of Human Genetics*, 56: 1493–1500.

Hietala, M., Aula, P., Syvänen, A-C., Isoniemi, A., Peltonen, L. and Palotie, A. (1996) 'DNA-based carrier screening in primary health care: screening for aspartylglucosaminuria in maternity health care offices', *Clinical Chemistry*, 42: 1398–1404.

Hietala, M., Hakonen, A., Aro, A.R., Niemelä, P., Peltonen, L. and Aula, P. (1998) 'Acceptance and experiences of carrier screening among Finnish pregnant women and primary care nurses: a pilot study using an aspartylglucosaminuria gene test', published as one of the original communications in M. Hietala, *Prospects for Genetic Screening in Finland*. Turku: University of Turku.

Ikonen, E. and Palotie, L. (1994) 'AGU-tauti: pistemutaatio kehitysvammaisuuden syynä', *Duodecim*, 110: 667–673.

Isoniemi, A., Hietala, M., Aula, P., Jalanko, A. and Peltonen, L. (1995) 'Identification of a novel mutation causing aspartylglucosaminuria reveals a mutation hotspot region in the aspartylglucosaminidase gene', *Human Mutation*, 5: 318–326.

Jallinoja, P. (2002) *Genetics, Negotiated Ethics and the Ambiguities of Moral Choices*. Helsinki: National Public Health Institute.

Jallinoja, P. and Aro, A.R. (2000) 'Does knowledge make a difference? The association between knowledge about genes and attitudes towards gene tests', *Journal of Health Communication*, 5: 29–39.

Jallinoja, P., Hakonen, A., Aro, A.R., Niemelä, P., Hietala, M., Lönnqvist, J., Peltonen, L. and Aula, P. (1998) 'Attitudes towards genetic testing: analysis of contradictions', *Social Science & Medicine*, 46: 1367–1374.

Naglie, G., Krahn, M.D., Naimark, D., Redelmeier, D.A. and Detsky, A.S. (1997) 'Primer on medical decision analysis, Part 3: estimating probabilities and utilities', *Medical Decision Making*, 17: 136–141.

Norio, R., Nevanlinna, H.R. and Perheentupa, J. (1973) 'Hereditary diseases in Finland: rare flora in rare soil', *Annals of Clinical Research*, 5: 109–141.

Novas, C. and Rose, N. (2000) 'Genetic risk and the birth of the somatic individual', *Economy and Society*, 29: 485–513.

O'Malley, P. (1996) 'Risk and responsibility', in A. Barry, T. Osborne and N. Rose (eds.) *Foucault and Political Reason: Liberalism, Neo-Liberalism and Rationalities of Government*. London: UCL Press.

Petersen, A. (1997) 'Risk, governance and the new public health', in A. Petersen and R. Bunton (eds.) *Foucault, Health and Medicine*. London and New York: Routledge.

Rose, N. (1998) *Inventing our Selves: Psychology, Power, and Personhood*. Cambridge and New York: Cambridge University Press.

Rose, N. (2001) 'The politics of life itself', *Theory, Culture & Society*, 18: 1–30.

Syvänen, A-C., Ikonen, E., Manninen, T., Bengtström, M., Söderlund, H., Aula, P. and Peltonen, L. (1992) 'Convenient and quantitative determination of the frequency of a mutant allele using solid-phase minisequencing: application to aspartylglucosaminuria in Finland', *Genomics*, 12: 590–595.

Teikari, M. (2003) 'Sikiöseulontaa tehostetaan Alankomaissa – seerumiseula käyttöön', *Impakti*, 1: 7–9.

Turner, B. S. (1997) 'Foreword: From governmentality to risk, some reflections on Foucault's contribution to medical sociology', in A. Petersen and R. Bunton (eds.) *Foucault, Health and Medicine*. London and New York: Routledge.

Ubel, P.A. and Loewenstein, G. (1997) 'The role of decision analysis in informed consent: choosing between intuition and systematicity', *Social Science & Medicine*, 44: 647–656.

Valkonen, S., Hietala, M., Savontaus, M-L. and Aula, P. (1999) 'Origin of Finnish mutations causing aspartylglucosaminuria', *Hereditas*, 131: 191–195.

Chapter 4

Choice as responsibility

Genetic testing as citizenship through familial obligation and the management of risk

Jessica Polzer

Introduction

Over the past two decades, the concept of 'risk' has become central to professional and non-professional understandings of health, and to the ways in which public health activities are organized and carried out, in Canada and elsewhere in the Western world (Bunton et al. 1994; Gabe 1995; Skolbekken 1995; Petersen and Lupton 1996). More recently, scientific knowledge of the genetic mutations implicated in the development of particular diseases has flourished, and consequently, our understandings of health risk are becoming 'geneticized' (Lippman 1991, 1994, 2000).

Discourses on risk and the new genetics converge in the practice of predictive genetic testing in which individuals with family histories that suggest an inherited form of disease can – with the provision of a blood sample – procure knowledge about their own susceptibility to the disease later in life. As genetic testing services for late-onset disorders become more widely available, there is a growing body of research that has examined genetic testing from the viewpoint of those being tested (Evans et al. 1994; Lerman et al. 1996; Lloyd et al. 1996; Chapple et al. 1997; Hallowell 1997; Jacobsen et al. 1997; Tambor et al. 1997; Marteau and Croyle 1998; Bluman et al. 1999; Cull et al. 1999; Lipkus et al. 1999; Warner et al. 1999; Watson et al. 1999). With some notable exceptions (Parsons and Atkinson 1992; Jallinoja et al. 1998; Cox and McKellin 1999; Hallowell 1999; Robertson 2000, 2001; Taylor 2004), a significant number of these studies have been concerned with judging the accuracy of lay perceptions compared to expert definitions of risk. While such studies provide insight into individuals' perceptions of health risks, by positioning 'lay people' as passive recipients of expert knowledge, this research forecloses a focus on how individuals actively participate in knowledge-making about their genetic risk, and how they come to understand their genetic risk in the context of their everyday lives. Furthermore, because this body of research tends to stay at the level of description, it is limited in its ability to provoke thought about how personal meanings and experiences of 'genetic risk' are embedded within, and connect up with, broader political arrangements and the public health practices these arrangements foster.

In this chapter, I use the theoretical lens of governmentality and the concept of citizenship in order to situate predictive genetic testing as a neoliberal technique of governance. After elaborating this theoretical position in the first section of the chapter, empirical data are presented as a case study to illustrate how individuals, through their participation in genetic testing, actively construct themselves as responsible citizens by fulfilling their duties to know and manage their genetic risk, and to inform their blood relatives of their potential genetic predisposition to disease so that they too can act as responsible risk managers. The implications of these findings are then discussed to consider how notions of 'choice', the 'carrier' and the 'family' are constituted and configured within discourses on genetic risk.

Genetic testing as a neoliberal technique of governance

A Foucauldian notion of governance, or governmentality, not only focuses on the workings of the state, but also includes a consideration of the entire set of practices involved in the 'conduct of conduct' – i.e. in the directing of human action towards particular goals or norms (Foucault 1991; Gordon 1991; Dean 1999). From this perspective, 'public health' is conceptualized as an assemblage of practices and expert knowledges that privilege particular types of subjects and establish norms for conduct in everyday life (e.g. Nettleton 1991, 1994; Lupton 1995; Gastaldo 1997; Petersen 1997, 1998, 1999; Howson 1998). As an assemblage of governmental practices, public health operates not only through state-directed regulatory strategies, but also by invoking individuals' desires to regulate their own conduct in the name of health.

From this point of view, it is possible to see how the knowledge forms and practices associated with the new genetics and with public health come together at various sites in the governance of both individuals and populations. Such practices of governance include activities carried out by the state (e.g. policy-making) and those of the biotechnology industry (e.g. in shaping biomedical research), the creation of knowledge about genetic norms and genetic risk (e.g. the Human Genome Project, epidemiological research), the translation of such knowledge into clinical practice (e.g. genetic testing clinics), the education and training of genetic specialists who advise individuals about their inherited susceptibility to disease (e.g. genetic counsellors) and the practices of self-governance by which individuals seek out and use genetic risk information to alter their own behaviours and their relationships with others (e.g. reproductive decision-making).

Whereas public health practices based on the 'old eugenics' mainly involved state-directed coercive regulatory strategies targeted at those judged to be genetically unfit (e.g. forced sterilization) in order to restrict their reproductive freedom, contemporary forms of genetic testing operate primarily as neoliberal techniques of governance in which experts (e.g. epidemiologists) define norms and act as advisers (e.g. genetic counsellors), yet which facilitate individual autonomy by encouraging individuals to take an active role in decision-making about genetic testing (Petersen 1997, 1999). In general, neoliberal programmes of governance include multiple practices and techniques that facilitate autonomous self-regulation and encourage individuals to make responsible choices for themselves and for those to whom they are socially and biologically connected (e.g. family, community) (Rose 1996a). The objectives of neoliberal governmental practices are thus achieved not through a repression of individuals' powers, but through the activation of individuals themselves to exercise their autonomy and freedom of choice in particular ways towards their own self-regulation (Miller and Rose 1994; Rose 1996b).

Neoliberal practices of governance utilize active citizenship as a key strategy by which this regulated autonomy is accomplished (Rose 1993, 1999; Petersen 1999, 2002). Discourses on genetic risk, informed by the imperatives of 'right to know' and 'informed choice' (Petersen 1998), invite individuals to exercise their right to know their genetic risk status so that they can make decisions about, and take charge of, their health in light of their inherited biological risks. This emphasis on informed decision-making presumes and operates through the agency of individuals themselves who are expected not only to exercise their rights to demand access to genetic testing services and to obtain knowledge about their genetic risk, but also to modify their lifestyles in light of their newly acquired knowledge of their inherent genetic risks. It is thus through the willingness of individuals themselves to take charge of their health that they are governed as neoliberal subjects, and through which they fulfil the obligations necessary to construct themselves as active, healthy and responsible citizens.

Using governmentality to understand individuals' experiences of genetic testing

The remainder of this chapter uses the notion of governmentality as an analytic lens to investigate empirically how individuals experience and understand their participation in genetic testing. The interview data presented in this section were drawn from a qualitative study that was conducted in 1999 to explore the perspectives of individuals attending a familial melanoma clinic in Ontario, Canada. At the time the study was conducted, the clinic operated for one half day per week and provided testing for genetic mutations (at p16, chromosome 9) associated with familial melanoma risk as part of a research project. The objectives of this study were to gather information about the knowledge, attitudes and beliefs that the clinic's attendees had regarding melanoma risk and prevention, and to explore the factors influencing their decision-making to attend the clinic and to accept or defer genetic testing. The overall aim of this pilot project was to develop a set of practice recommendations for the clinic based on what was learned from the interviews with the genetic testing participants.

Semi-structured interviews were conducted with twenty-seven individuals who were referred to the clinic, who were at various stages in the process of genetic testing, and who met the clinic referral criteria of having at least one relative (living or deceased) with a diagnosis of malignant melanoma. Interviews were audio-recorded and transcribed verbatim, which produced approximately one thousand pages of qualitative data. Data analysis was conducted using an adaptation of the method of constant comparisons (Glaser and Strauss 1967; Strauss and Corbin 1990) which involved generating descriptive codes that were grounded in respondents' accounts. Descriptive codes were then combined into broader, analytic themes developed by the analyst to represent the ways in which respondents conceptualized the responsibilities they associated with their participation in genetic testing. Data analysis was conducted with the assistance of the NUD*IST 4.0 computerized qualitative data analysis software (Richards and Richards 1996). The quotes included here have been chosen on the basis of their clarity and ability to illustrate these analytic themes, and pseudonyms have been assigned to the study participants to protect their anonymity.

Results

Three analytic themes are used to present the duties and responsibilities that the study participants associated with their decision-making regarding genetic testing: the duty to know genetic risk, the duty to manage genetic risk and the duty to inform family members of inherited risk. Participants' accounts were surprisingly similar with respect to these analytic themes, regardless of where they were at in the process of genetic testing. Some differences were observed, however, between the accounts of participants who had been affected with melanoma and those who had never been diagnosed with melanoma. Where relevant, these differences have been noted.

The duty to know genetic risk: 'being aware'

In general, participants felt that obtaining information about the risk factors and signs of melanoma would facilitate the early detection of a malignancy. In general, respondents felt that 'the more information one had about their health, the better' because this would instil a greater 'awareness' of health risks and of bodily signs of normality and abnormality (i.e. irregular moles). Specifically, the process of genetic testing was seen to influence the ways in which the study participants examined their bodies for signs of potential cancer by heightening their awareness of the shapes and configurations of 'healthy' and 'unhealthy' moles. For example, when asked whether she viewed herself differently in light of her positive test result, Dawn, who had been diagnosed with melanoma already, responded:

> I find I'm looking closer at things that I didn't look at before . . . I think that I'm . . . more clinically observant. I'm not just seeing a mole any longer and going 'Oh yeah, another mole'. I'm more aware of the configurations of things and I'm looking in more obscure places.
>
> (Dawn, had previous melanoma)

This heightened clinical awareness of bodily signs of normality and abnormality was seen by participants as crucial to optimize the chances of early detection and to avoid the development of malignant skin cancer and invasive surgical treatment. Whereas participants who already had melanoma were in the routine of doing regular skin examinations, for the unaffected individuals, obtaining knowledge of genetic risk was seen as particularly important to improve their chances of early detection through the effects this knowledge would have on intensifying medical and self-surveillance:

> It's [genetic testing] another set of eyes. Like my impression is I'm in a relatively high-risk [group] and the more people who are looking the more likely that it will get caught in plenty of time so that it's not a major issue.
>
> (George, no previous melanoma)

The duty to manage genetic risk: 'taking an active role in health'

Obtaining genetic risk information was framed by the study participants as an important step that would enable them to consider how they could adjust the preventive actions in which they were already engaged, and thus to plan for their futures. This was a strong theme in all the interviews and reflected the imperative for individuals to manage their genetic risk, primarily through increased surveillance and lifestyle modifications. Thus, the desire expressed by participants to 'be aware' of their genetic risk was intrinsically tied to the actions they took towards their future health on the basis of that information. Dorothy, who received a positive test result, describes this intrinsic connection:

> for some people just having the knowledge that that [melanoma] is a potential problem could make them more cautious – could make them more

> aware of what their potential risks are and maybe they can do a little bit more in the prevention and early detection side.
>
> (Dorothy, previous melanoma)

The framing of genetic risk information as constituting an initial step towards the prevention of melanoma was especially salient for those who had not been diagnosed with melanoma previously and/or who were not engaging in regular medical surveillance for melanoma. In the following passage, Susan clearly describes how genetic risk information would enable her to plan for her health in the future:

> the more information that you've got the better. As I said, some people, that can really bother them . . . stress them out a little bit. But I believe that if you know anything that's there then it can help you plan for the future . . . being examined more or if you have to change your lifestyle depending upon what you've been told [about the test results].
>
> (Susan, no previous melanoma)

Even some of the participants who refused testing could understand how genetic risk information could enable them to be more proactive in their own health, as this information would allow them to target their preventive actions more specifically depending on the types of biological risks they had inherited:

> I think that we need to take an active role in our own health by getting as much information as we can . . . It helps you to prepare. It helps you to know what you can do specifically. I think there are people who are fearful of getting cancer in general, all different kinds of cancer so they either do whatever they can in preventing it and do everything for every type of cancer, when in fact wouldn't it be nice to know for that person that they really should be concentrating on a particular type of cancer?
>
> (Nicole, no previous melanoma)

The duty to inform family members of inherited risk: genetic testing as familial obligation

In their accounts of why they decided to consider or undergo genetic testing, interview participants expressed a strong obligation to 'pass along' genetic risk information to their family members. It was felt that, through this communication of health risk information, family members would not only gain an awareness of their possible inherited predisposition to melanoma, but they would also be motivated to learn how to recognize bodily signs of potential disease (i.e. irregular moles) and to be more vigilant regarding self- and medical surveillance in order to detect a melanoma in its earliest stages of development:

> You're doing it [getting tested] so that your family has the information and you can prepare . . . it just makes them aware that it's a possibility and in order to keep themselves healthy they have to be aware of their bodies. They have to watch for signs and they have to take steps to try to protect themselves.
>
> (Melissa, previous melanoma)

Because they were already engaged in regular self- and medical surveillance, respondents who had already been affected with melanoma focused more on the benefits of testing for their family members than for themselves. Acquiring genetic risk information for one's children was seen as a particularly important responsibility among these study participants. However, responsibility to inform siblings and extended family members, and to encourage them to engage in greater self-surveillance, was also evident in the participants' accounts:

> I think [a positive test result] would certainly make them [my relatives] more aware and probably get them more into the sort of self checking mode . . . I think about nieces and nephews who are at the 'party in the sun' age so it may have more of an impact on them than probably us so . . .
>
> (Mike, no previous melanoma)

Similarly, participation in genetic testing was seen as having the potential to help future family members 'down the line' indirectly through the advancement of medical knowledge. For Susan, who received a negative test result, this perceived benefit outweighed any negative consequences that a positive test result may have had for her personally:

> Well, my choice is can I help my family? . . . I mean my family meaning all the way down the line. You know, can I do something to help? Then yeah, I'm going to do it. It may give me knowledge that I may or may not have wanted to have, but now will have to deal with, but that's life. Sometimes you don't have the knowledge you need and sometimes you have knowledge you wish you didn't.
>
> (Susan, no previous melanoma)

To summarize, in addition to the implications that testing had for managing their own genetic risk, participants also felt a responsibility to gain knowledge of their genetic risk so that this information could be 'carried forward' to their children, to their more extended family members, and to future family members. Through the acquisition and provision of genetic risk information, participants felt that their relatives would be able to gain a greater awareness of their bodies, and would be encouraged to be more vigilant in their strategies to manage their risk for familial melanoma.

Doing the right thing? Ambivalence about 'carrying' genetic risk information

While participants' accounts were strongly shaped by the responsibility they felt to provide family members with genetic risk information, a minority of the study participants were clearly ambivalent about this 'duty to inform'. For these individuals, information about genetic risk was a double-edged sword. On the one hand, the provision of genetic risk information was seen as encouraging family members to be more aware of their bodies, and to be more vigilant in their skin surveillance and sun protection practices. On the other hand, it was felt that genetic risk information might provoke in their children and other relatives undue fear, anxiety and a sense of wariness towards their own bodies. This ambivalence was particularly strong among those individuals who had already had melanoma and who were engaged in regular skin surveillance strategies, for they felt that they were already communicating preventive messages to their children and other family members. A mother whose children had witnessed her experiences with melanoma expresses this tension in the following passage:

> . . . it's education being a protection as opposed to a hindrance. I think that whole concept is where it's at but it's also very scary. And what do you do with that information once you have it? Yes I think it would be a good thing to know. I could come home and say to the family, 'Okay, I have this in my DNA and chances are you do too and you have to watch for it'. The thing is I've already done that in a sense. You know they've watched me go through my own melanoma journey and we've discussed the fact that this can happen to anybody . . . on the one hand you want to keep the fear out of it, you don't want to make them afraid, but at the same time you want to make them aware.
>
> (Melissa, previous melanoma)

In a different vein, the ambivalence of some participants towards the communication of genetic risk information to their children was rooted in their belief that health is not exclusively a matter of personal choice or self-control. This father is clearly of two minds when he simultaneously acknowledges the potential value of genetic risk information in informing his children's health practices, yet firmly maintains his belief that the future is often beyond individual control:

> perhaps it'll be in the forefront that they'll take better care of their health, their bodies . . . but I would stress to them that you really cannot change what's going to happen to you – I mean, if I get it [melanoma] you have to deal with that. If they get it [melanoma] we all have to deal with it. I mean, they have their life to live. So do I . . . you really have no control over a lot

> of things in your life and that's one of the things, so you just gotta go on. I mean, you can't let it dictate to you what you're going to do or how you're going to do it or when you're going to do it.
>
> (Tom, no previous melanoma)

Discussion

Using the analytic lens of governmentality, I have argued that genetic testing constitutes one site for the construction and exercise of citizenship in which individuals willingly acquire information about their genetic risk to facilitate and direct their own health-related actions, as well as those of their current and future family members. Specifically, this study illustrates how the practice of predictive genetic testing invokes three interrelated duties or responsibilities: the duty to acquire genetic risk information to facilitate bodily awareness, increased surveillance, and the early detection of disease; the duty to engage in more precise risk management on the basis of one's knowledge of their genetic susceptibility to disease; and the duty to communicate one's genetic risk status to family members. It is through this participation in genetic testing and the fulfilment of these duties that individuals can construct themselves as healthy and responsible citizens – doing all they can to 'arm' themselves and their family members with the information they see as necessary to manage their health risks and to ward off the threat of disease.

That these duties were taken up so willingly by the participants in this study attests to the power of predictive genetic testing to facilitate particular forms of citizenship in which individuals are encouraged to take responsibility for their own health by managing their relationship to their biologically inherited risk (Petersen 2002). The results of this study suggest that genetic testing is seen by individuals to provide them with the information they need to plan their futures and inform the 'choices' they make (e.g. lifestyle modifications, increased screening) in order to maintain their health and that of their family members. By situating genetic testing as a neoliberal technique of governance, it is possible to problematize this notion of 'informed choice' both as an objective and as a benefit of genetic testing. This is not to suggest that individuals should necessarily have more or less choice concerning their access to and participation in emerging genetic services such as predictive genetic testing. Rather, the point to be emphasized here is that it is precisely through their participation in genetic testing that individuals come to recognize what their choices are, make decisions based on those choices, and simultaneously learn how to conduct their lives and regulate their behaviours in ways suggested by their newly acquired knowledge of their biologically inherited risks. In other words, as a neoliberal technique of governance, predictive genetic testing privileges a particular configuration between 'choice' and 'regulation' such that individuals perform their freedom in ways that cast them as responsible citizens who actively take charge of their health through personal and familial risk management.

By locating risk within one's genetic make-up, this regulated autonomy is accomplished through predictive genetic testing by constructing individuals not only as *harbourers* of mutated genes (who are called upon to tailor their risk-reduction strategies to minimize the likelihood of disease), but also as *carriers* of mutated genes. Furthermore, in so far as individuals understand their involvement in genetic testing as influenced by their desire to communicate genetic risk information to family members, they actively construct themselves as *carriers of health risk information*. This dual construction of 'the carrier', in terms of both biological information *and* health risk information, effectively translates embodied genetic risks into personal and social responsibilities.

By showing how study participants constructed themselves as 'carriers' of health risk information, this study illustrates the specific ways in which predictive genetic testing constitutes the family as the 'natural link' between the personal ethic of maintaining good health and more general political objectives (Foucault 1977, 1991; Petersen and Lupton 1996). The establishment of risk within a web of 'genetic connectedness' (Novas and Rose 2000) demarcates 'the family' as a territory of government in which the family is constructed as both an object of, and a vehicle for, genetic governance. As this and other studies have shown (e.g. Hallowell 1999), the welfare of one's relatives often factors into decision-making about whether or not to undergo genetic testing for cancer risk. To the extent that genetic testing recipients feel responsible in communicating genetic risk information to their family members, individuals themselves become instrumental in the deployment of knowledge concerning genetic risk. It is through this 'duty to inform' that individuals become active not only in their own self-governance, but also in the governance of their biological relatives. This relational aspect of genetic risk is significant, for individuals may agree to genetic testing for the sake of their family members even if they do not see any personal benefits (Hallowell 1999). In this way, by invoking one's duty to inform family members about genetic risk, the practice of genetic testing is further implicated in the 'conduct of conduct' – or in the regulation of freedom – by constraining one's choice to refuse knowledge about their genetic risk.

While the responsibility to transmit genetic risk information to family members was a strong theme, adoption of this carrier subject was contested by some of the participants in this study. These individuals did not dismiss the idea of genetic testing altogether, but were clearly ambivalent about the effects that genetic risk information might have on their family members, particularly their children. This ambivalence, or contradiction in attitudes, toward genetic testing has been reported elsewhere (Jallinoja et al. 1998) and can be understood using the theoretical perspective employed in this chapter. That is, individuals who resist the role of risk information carrier place themselves in a precarious position because if they want to protect their family members from what they see as potentially anxiety-provoking information about their inherited risk, they must do so at the cost of being able to fulfil the obligations necessary to construct themselves as responsible citizens.

Conclusion

Through the analytic lens of governmentality, we can see how the 'choices' brought into view by emerging genetic technologies, and individuals' experiences of those technologies, are produced within, and contingent upon, a neoliberal vision of public health that is achieved through the individual (informed) actions of citizens who take responsibility for their health by engaging in various practices (e.g. genetic testing, lifestyle modifications) in order to manage their relationship to risk. By grounding this theoretical stance in individuals' own experiences of emerging genetic technologies, we can see more closely how neoliberal techniques of governance operate – although not always successfully – *through the agency of individuals themselves* as they actively work to cultivate their own bodies and everyday lives to reduce cancer-related risks and disseminate health risk information to their family members. While the practices of genetic testing and counselling purport to facilitate 'autonomy' over decision-making (Petersen 2002), this study showed that decision-making is not always straightforward – individuals often overlook their own choice not to know genetic risk information for the sake of their family's health, and they sometimes grapple with the difficulties of deciding whether or not they want their own children to have knowledge of their inherited potential for cancer.

As research on the personal, social and ethical implications of predictive genetic testing grows, Foucauldian-inspired and other types of critical analyses of 'real life' situations can help us to elucidate the ways in which the concepts of 'choice' and 'autonomy' are intrinsically connected to, and thus shaped by, individual experiences of familial obligation and responsible, active citizenship. Following the examples of other critical theorists (e.g. Lippman 2000; Robertson 2001; Sherwin 2001) such analyses might further question and critically appraise, for example: the specific ways in which the concepts of 'choice' and 'autonomy' are articulated through emerging genetic technologies to sustain individualist visions of health; whether or not these concepts are appropriate or desirable as objectives of predictive genetic testing which can yield uncertain and inconclusive test results; how these concepts are used to justify state investment in the biotechnology industry alongside the increasing marketization of health; and at what cost to the public's health is it justifiable to focus on, and invest resources in, the production of knowledge of the molecular mechanisms of disease.

Acknowledgements

Drs Vivek Goel and Shawna L. Mercer are gratefully acknowledged for their feedback, encouragement and support. This research was generously supported by a grant from the Medical Research Council of Canada.

References

Bluman, L.G., Rimer, B.K., Berry, D.A., Borstelmann, N., Iglehart, J.D., Regan, K., Schildkraut, J. and Winer, E.P. (1999) 'Attitudes, knowledge, and risk perceptions of women with breast and/or ovarian cancer considering testing for BRCA1 and BRCA2', *Journal of Clinical Oncology,* 19(3): 1040–1046.

Bunton, R., Nettleton, S. and Burrows, R. (1994) *The Sociology of Health Promotion: Critical Analyses of Consumption, Lifestyle and Risk*. London: Routledge.

Chapple, A., Campion, P. and May, C. (1997) 'Clinical terminology: anxiety and confusion amongst families undergoing genetic counseling', *Patient Education and Counseling*, 32: 81–91.

Cox, S. and McKellin, W. (1999) '"There's this thing in our family": predictive testing and the construction of risk for Huntington Disease', *Sociology of Health and Illness*, 21(5): 622–646.

Cull, A., Anderson, E.D., Campbell, S., Mackay, J., Smyth, E. and Steel, M. (1999) 'The impact of genetic counselling about breast cancer risk on women's risk perceptions and levels of distress', *British Journal of Cancer*, 79(3–4): 501–508.

Dean, M. (1999) *Governmentality: Power and Rule in Modern Society*. London: Sage.

Evans, D.G.R., Blair, V., Greenhalgh, R., Hopwood, P. and Howell, A. (1994) 'The impact of genetic counselling on risk perception in women with a family history of breast cancer', *British Journal of Cancer*, 74: 934–938.

Foucault, M. (1977) 'The politics of health in the eighteenth century', in C. Gordon (ed.) *Power/Knowledge: Selected Interviews and Other Writings, 1972–1977*. New York: Pantheon.

Foucault, M. (1991) 'Governmentality', in G. Burchell, C. Gordon and P. Miller (eds) *The Foucault Effect: Studies in Governmentality*. Hemel Hempstead: Harvester Wheatsheaf.

Gabe, J. (1995) 'Health, medicine and risk: the need for a sociological approach', in J. Gabe (ed.) *Medicine, Health and Risk: Sociological Approaches*. Oxford: Blackwell.

Gastaldo, D. (1997) 'Is health education good for you? Rethinking health education through the concept of bio-power', in A. Petersen and R. Bunton (eds) *Foucault, Health and Medicine*. London: Routledge.

Glaser, B.G. and Strauss, A.L. (1967) *The Discovery of Grounded Theory: Strategies for Qualitative Research*. Chicago: Aldine.

Gordon, C. (1991) 'Governmental rationality: an introduction', in G. Burchell, C. Gordon and P. Miller (eds) *The Foucault Effect: Studies in Governmentality*. Chicago: University of Chicago Press.

Hallowell, N. (1997) 'Understanding life's lottery: an evaluation of studies of genetic risk awareness', *Journal of Health Psychology*, 2(1): 31–43.

Hallowell, N. (1999) 'Doing the right thing: genetic risk and responsibility', *Sociology of Health and Illness*, 21(5): 597–621.
Howson, A. (1998) 'Embodied obligation: the female body and health surveillance', in S. Nettleton and J. Watson (eds) *The Body in Everyday Life*. London: Routledge.
Jacobsen, P.B., Valdimarsdottier, H.B., Brown, K.L. and Offit, K. (1997) 'Decision-making about genetic testing among women at familial risk for breast cancer', *Psychosomatic Medicine*, 59(5): 459–466.
Jallinoja, P., Hakonen, A., Aro, A.R., Niemela, M., Hietala, M., Lonnqvist, J., Peltonen, L. and Aula, P. (1998) 'Attitudes towards genetic testing: analysis of contradictions', *Social Science and Medicine*, 46(10): 1367–1374.
Lerman, C., Marshall, J., Audrain, J. and Gomez-Caminero, A. (1996) 'Genetic testing for colon cancer susceptibility: anticipated reactions of patients and challenges to providers', *International Journal of Cancer*, 69: 58–61.
Lipkus, I.M., Iden, D., Terrenoire, J. and Feaganes, J.R. (1999) 'Relationships among breast cancer concern, risk perceptions, and interest in genetic testing for breast cancer susceptibility among African-American women with and without a family history of breast cancer', *Cancer Epidemiological Biomarkers Prevention*, 8(6): 533–539.
Lippman, A. (1991) 'Prenatal genetic testing and screening: constructing needs and reinforcing inequities', *American Journal of Law and Medicine*, 17(1–2): 15–50.
Lippman, A. (1994) 'Worrying – and worrying about – the geneticization of reproduction and health', in G. Basen, M. Eichler and A. Lippman (eds) *Misconceptions: The Social Construction of Choice and the New Reproductive and Genetic Technologies*. Prescott, ON: Voyageur.
Lippman, A. (2000) 'Geneticization and the Canadian Biotechnology Strategy: the marketing of women's health', in *The Gender of Genetic Futures: The Canadian Biotechnology Strategy, Women and Health*. Proceedings of a National Strategic Workshop, York University, Toronto, February.
Lloyd, S., Watson, M., Waites, B., Meyer, L., Eeles, R., Ebbs, S. and Tylee, A. (1996) 'Familial breast cancer: a controlled study of risk perception, psychological morbidity and health beliefs in women attending for genetic counselling', *British Journal of Cancer*, 74(3): 482–487.
Lupton, D. (1995) *The Imperative of Health: Public Health and the Regulated Body*. London: Sage.
Marteau, T. and Croyle, R.T. (1998) 'Psychological responses to genetic testing', *British Medical Journal*, 316: 693–696.
Miller, P. and Rose, N. (1994) 'On therapeutic authority: psychoanalytical expertise under advanced liberalism', *History of the Human Sciences*, 7(3): 29–64.
Nettleton, S. (1991) 'Wisdom, diligence and teeth: discursive practices and the creation of mothers', *Sociology of Health and Illness*, 13(1): 98–111.
Nettleton, S. (1994) 'Disciplinary power and dentistry', in C. Jones and R. Porter (eds) *Reassessing Foucault: Power, Medicine and the Body*. London: Routledge.
Novas, C. and Rose, N. (2000) 'Genetic risk and the birth of the somatic individual', *Economy and Society*, 29(4): 485–513.
Parsons, E. and Atkinson, P. (1992) 'Lay constructions of genetic risk', *Sociology of Health and Illness*, 14(4): 437–455.
Petersen, A. (1997) 'Risk, governance and the new public health', in A. Petersen and R. Bunton (eds) *Foucault, Health and Medicine*. London: Routledge.

Petersen, A. (1998) 'The new genetics and the politics of public health', *Critical Public Health*, 8(1): 59–71.

Petersen, A. (1999) 'Public health, the new genetics and subjectivity', in A. Petersen, I. Barns, J. Dudley and P. Harris (eds) *Poststructuralism, Citizenship and Social Policy*. London: Routledge.

Petersen, A. (2002) 'Facilitating autonomy: the discourse of genetic counselling', in A. Petersen and R. Bunton (eds) *The New Genetics and the Public's Health*. London: Routledge.

Petersen, A. and Lupton, D. (1996) *The New Public Health: Health and Self in the Age of Risk*. London: Sage.

Richards, L. and Richards, T. (1996) *QSR NUD*IST (Non numerical Unstructured Data Indexing Searching and Theory-building) (Version 4.0)*. Sydney: Qualitative Solutions & Research.

Robertson, A. (2000) 'Embodying risk, embodying political rationality: women's accounts of risks for breast cancer', *Health, Risk and Society*, 2(2): 219–235.

Robertson, A. (2001) 'Biotechnology, political rationality and discourses on health risk', *Health*, 5(3): 293–309.

Rose, N. (1993) 'Government, authority and expertise in advanced liberalism', *Economy and Society*, 22(3): 283–299.

Rose, N. (1996a) 'The death of the social? Re-figuring the territory of government', *Economy and Society*, 25(3): 327–356.

Rose, N. (1996b) 'Governing "advanced" liberal democracies', in A. Barry, T. Osborne and N. Rose (eds) *Foucault and Political Reason: Liberalism, Neoliberalism and Rationalities of Government*. Chicago: University of Chicago Press.

Rose, N. (1999) *Powers of Freedom: Reframing Political Thought*. Cambridge: Cambridge University Press.

Sherwin, S. (2001) *Towards an Adequate Ethical Framework for Setting Biotechnology Policy*. Prepared for the Canadian Biotechnology Advisory Committee Stewardship Standing Committee, http://strategis.ic.gc.ca/epic/internet/incbac-cccb.nsf/en/ah0040e.html (accessed 26 October 2004).

Skolbekken, J. (1995) 'The risk epidemic in medical journals', *Social Science and Medicine*, 40(3): 291–305.

Strauss, A. and Corbin, J. (1990) *Basics of Qualitative Research: Grounded Theory Procedures and Techniques*. Newbury Park, CA: Sage.

Tambor, E.S., Rimer, B.K. and Strigo, T.S. (1997) 'Genetic testing for breast cancer susceptibility: awareness and interest among women in the general population', *American Journal of Medical Genetics*, 68(1): 43–49.

Taylor, S. (2004) 'Predictive genetic test decisions for Huntington's disease: context, appraisal and new moral imperatives', *Social Science & Medicine*, 58: 137–149.

Warner, E., Heisey, R.E., Goel, V., Carroll, J.C. and McCready, D.R. (1999) 'Hereditary breast cancer: risk assessment of patients with a family history of breast cancer', *Canadian Family Physician*, 45(January): 104–112.

Watson, M., Lloyd, S., Davidson, J., Meyer, L., Eeles, R., Ebbs, S. and Murday, V. (1999) 'The impact of genetic counselling on risk perception and mental health in women with a family history of breast cancer', *British Journal of Cancer*, 79(5–6): 868–874.

Part II

Risk, population and identity

Chapter 5

From eugenics to the government of genetic risks

Thomas Lemke

> ... we should not underestimate the dangers of a new eugenics. If biological tests are used to conform people to rigid institutional norms, we risk reducing social tolerance for the variation in human experience. We risk increasingly the number of people defined as unemployable, uneducable, or insurable. We risk creating a new biological underclass.
>
> (Nelkin and Tancredi 1994: 176)

Introduction

In the ongoing discussion about the social and ethical impact of genetic testing the question of eugenics is a central issue. At the heart of these debates is the fear that there will be a re-emergence, return or a 'backdoor to eugenics' (Duster 2003). Many critics regard contemporary medical genetic practices as a continuation of population policy, social cleansing and racist programmes such as were practised during the first half of the twentieth century in their most violent and brutal form by the Nazis. Conversely, most geneticists dissociate present medical genetics from these practices since they employ a narrow definition that identifies eugenics with coercion and repression. In their view there is a fundamental rupture between past eugenics and contemporary medical genetics since the latter relies on consensus and choice.

In the following, I propose to displace this debate by introducing the notion of governmentality as developed by the French philosopher and historian Michel Foucault. Foucault defines government in a very broad sense as conduct or, more precisely, as 'the conduct of conduct'; the term in Foucault's use refers to all endeavours to guide and direct the government of others, but it also includes forms of subjectivation: the government of the self (Foucault 1982a: 220–221, 1991; Lemke 1997). The analytics of governmentality links political strategies to the subject's capacity to govern itself and the mobilization of truth to the production of particular moral subject positions. Following Foucault, I am interested in how genetic knowledge and genetic technologies are used in the government of individuals and populations, how medical practices and diagnostic tools function as political technologies on the one hand and as moral technologies on the other hand.

As a consequence, the key point here is less whether contemporary medical genetics is eugenic or not, and more what we exactly mean by 'eugenics' today. By eugenics we used to understand 'the cluster of ideas and activities that aimed at improving the quality of the human race through the manipulation of its biological heredity' (Kevles 1992: 4).[1] To what contemporary fears and foreseeable future developments does this label refer? What parallels and what differences in present human genetic practices can be discerned compared, for example, with the Nazi racist project or the US sterilization programmes at the beginning of the twentieth century? In other words, the question concerns the historico-political continuities and ruptures between 'old' and 'new eugenics' (Proctor 1992; Paul 1994, 1998).

Medical genetics and eugenics: continuity or discontinuity?

When attempting to answer this question I proceed from a working hypothesis which proposes two lines demarcating the analysis: on the one hand, we cannot assume a more or less linear continuity of eugenic practices from the Nazis to the present. For this reason, I find it problematical to speak of 'old eugenics in a new guise' (Weikert 1998: 146), of a continuation of 'eugenic traditions on a higher technical level' (Schumann 1992: 62) or a 'relapse into biologistic patterns' (Koechlin 1996: 35). On the other, it is also not tenable to assume there has been a fundamental rupture between the old eugenics and current medical genetics. Such a hypothesis relies on scientific improvements in molecular genetics declaring eugenic goals to be obsolete as a result of new scientific findings. They point to the fact that research in genetics showed that mutations and genetic anomalies are a widespread phenomenon in a population that renders senseless the project of 'purification' or 'amelioration' of the gene pool (Propping 1992: 125–127; Winnacker 1997: 143–148). Another line of argumentation appeals to changes in 'motivational structures' (Junker and Paul 1999; see also Wolff 1990). The claim is that there could no longer be any talk of eugenics if individual decisions on reproduction geared to self-determined options and the principle of voluntary choice take the place of collective concern for the gene pool or the project of an evolutionary improvement in humanity. Let us consider the two positions one after the other.

As regards the *continuity hypothesis*, it has to be remembered that nature today can no longer be regarded as some immutable constant, unlike during the first half of the twentieth century and the heyday of eugenics. It is problematic to claim that the recourse to heredity simply replaces the discourse of environment, shifting the attention from one side to the other side of the nature–nurture debate. Rather, the new genetics displaces the two poles that once constituted the debate itself. Today, molecular biology and genetic engineering function as informational sciences, regarding the DNA as a code that can be read and rewritten (Kay 2000). As a result, the status of biology and the relation between biology and society is changed. It is therefore insufficient to state or to criticize the 'biologization of society', since the results of social science studies show that the dichotomy between nature and culture is itself getting more and more problematic (Haraway 1991; Keller 1992; Latour 1993).[2]

The identification of individuals with genetic risks does not serve to pinpoint some ineluctably biological fate; nor does it signify something which is beyond control. On the contrary, it refers to a privileged field of interventions. Like environmental risks, genetic risks could be calculated, but – in contrast to the former – they appear to be easier to measure and to control. Genetic diagnosis offers a series of possible interventions to avoid or minimize risk. These cover such different strategies as taking medicines and psychopharmaceuticals, the use of genetic therapies or the control of lifestyles, choice of partner, reproduction decisions, etc. In this respect, the significance of genetic diagnostics is above all in monitoring the potentially infirm and controlling the factors which could lead to the emergence of pathological states. The introduction and spread of genetic tests will dramatically improve the scope of information available for those who wish to enhance their 'quality of life' by avoiding illness and deviance from the norms:

> The logical progression of this type of development is a situation in which it would become common for people to know about their own genetic risk profile across a range of disorders, and for them to design an 'individually tailored' set of behaviours. Someone with an inherited susceptibility to coronary thrombosis and musculo-skeletal problems, for example, may decide never to eat high-fat foods nor play impact or contact sports. Another person with a quite different 'genetic read-out' may become particularly wary of entering smoky rooms, or being exposed to bright sunlight.
>
> (Davison 1996: 321–322; see also Rose 2000)

Let us go on to the second position, namely the *assumption of a discontinuity* between eugenics and human genetics. With the erosion of the borderline between nature and society and new biotechnological possibilities for the diagnosis of the genetic composition of individuals, the problem of eugenics does not disappear but on the contrary it becomes inescapable. Paradoxically, it is exactly the fact that reproduction by means of the new biotechnologies becomes the object of free decision-making and individual planning that makes this society inevitably eugenic:

> The genetic manipulation of humans confuses the spheres of freedom and necessity. The freedom to manipulate nature, providing copies or designing

> human beings following genetic blue prints produces at the same time the necessity to ascribe even our non-manipulated existence to a decision.
>
> (Nassehi 1998: 57, translated by TL)

Whether we like it or not, even the seemingly 'non-eugenic' decision against genetic diagnostics and selective abortion has a eugenic quality, since it is based on a (normative) decision: the decision that it is better not to decide. The choice of a 'natural' genetic make-up for an individual is only one option and one 'selection' among others, in any case it is an option – neither fate nor unchangeable (Kitcher 1996: 196–197).

Risk discourse and genetic testing

It has been well documented that the notion of risk occupies a central place in professional medical literature (Skolbekken 1995), in health policy documents (Hayes 1992) and in the new public health (Petersen and Lupton 1996). Genetic risk has recently become equally important. My own research shows that the number of medical articles that deal with the term 'genetic risk(s)' in the title or abstract of the MEDLINE database increased rapidly from the end of the 1960s to the beginning of the new millennium. While only 4 articles are listed for the period from 1967 to 1971, ten years later 67 'genetic risk' articles were published (1977–1981); another ten years later the count is 211 (1987–1991), while it goes up to 1082 for the period from 1997 to 2001. The strategic concentration on genetic risks in medical research and clinical practice is also visible in the two application areas for genetic testing.

At present the main application area is that of prenatal diagnostics (and – to a lesser extent – preimplantation diagnostics). Under the sign of genetic testing, any pregnancy virtually becomes a 'risk pregnancy' or 'tentative pregnancy' (Rothman 1987), whereby allowing the embryo to live depends on the result of a test that rules out genetic abnormalities. The proclaimed privacy of each individual's decision and the decriminalization of abortion contrasts with the public pressure to (re)produce 'normal' children. The pregnant woman is conceived of not only as two people, but also as two patients with separate or even hostile interests. She is called on to work actively to optimize the foetus' health – and to avoid anything that could damage it. If, on the one hand, the woman (e.g. through claims for damages filed against the doctors responsible) is guaranteed a right to a healthy (i.e. 'undamaged') child, then, on the other, she is degraded to the status of 'foetal environment' which should engage in risk-minimizing behaviour (Steinberg 1996; Weir 1996; see also Ruhl 1999).

It is foreseeable that in the future the focus of genetic testing procedures might shift to persons already born (postnatal diagnostics). While genetic testing in this area was primarily used to detect very rare disorders, the decoding of the human genome and the isolation of genes that are associated with common diseases like cancer or heart disease raise the possibility of providing predictive information to many more people. Although in most cases genetic diagnostic procedures do not enable one to predict with certainty whether a person will develop a certain disease in the future they have already contributed to producing a new category of subjects: individuals 'at risk' (Billings et al. 1992; see Kenen 1996) who in the framework of genetic examinations and tests have been diagnosed to run the risk of certain illnesses which they may perhaps or may not possibly contract in the future. As surveys in several countries have shown, these 'risk individuals' or 'asymptomatic ill' are already confronted with real forms of genetic discrimination in the present. The perceived genetic variation from the 'normal' human genotype may result in forms of stigmatization and exclusion that range from a denial of insurance coverage to employment difficulties (Billings et al. 1992; Low et al. 1998; Thébaud Mondy 1999).

The risk discourse does not depend on the authority of the state but on the autonomy of the individual. Instead of eugenic programmes enforced by state institutions, relying primarily on repressive means, we observe today apparatuses of risk, aiming at the productive enhancement of the individual human capital in the name of self-determination and choice. A pluralism of authorities induces and encourages individuals to take responsibility for their own decisions concerning health and reproduction. Health experts and bioethicists teach and persuade us to make 'rational' and 'informed' choices that are based on genetic knowledge. They claim that genetic factors regulate or influence important diseases of civilization like obesity, cancer, schizophrenia, depression, Alzheimer's disease, diabetes, high blood pressure and coronary heart diseases (Clark 1997; Wertz et al. 2003). Medical advice literature reminds its readers that their 'genetic destiny' is in their own hands. Here the right for health gives place to an imperative to get as informed as possible about genetic risks:

> Know your family history, be cognizant of your ethnic origin, determine your genetic susceptibilities, opt for necessary gene tests, take preventive actions, establish appropriate surveillance, and seek preemptive treatment where applicable. In this way, you can exercise control over your genetic destiny, secure your health, and – in more ways than you yet realize – save your life.
>
> (Milunsky 2001: xv; see also Teichler-Zallen 1997; Bland and Benum 1999)

Genetic responsibility and the government of the self

Genome analysis and genetic diagnostics do rely less on a deterministic relationship between genes and diseases but generate a 'reflexive' relationship between individual risk profiles and social requirements (Lemke 2004). The reference to personal responsibility and self-determination in the biosciences makes sense only if the individual is more than a victim or prisoner of her or his genetic material. He or she is conceived not as a passive recipient of medical advice, but as an active seeker of information and consumer of genetic testing devices and health care services (Petersen and Bunton 2002). This strategy produces and exploits the imagery that future diseases, disorders and disabilities can be foretold and prevented by examining the individual genome. If indeed there were a direct relationship between genotype and phenotype in the sense of genetic determinism, then it would be more difficult to uphold the appeal to individual autonomy. By contrast, the construction of risk individuals, risk couples, risk pregnancies, etc. makes it easier to moralize on deviant behaviour and to assign guilt and responsibility (Douglas 1990). The definition of risk spaces enables therapies and forms of prevention to come to bear in a non-medical and a supra-individual sense and raises predictive genetic diagnostics to the status of a social medicine (Rose 2001).

The concept of information is crucial in this context since it serves simultaneously as the 'code of life' and as the 'key to freedom'. If the body is nothing other than a genetic programme, then disease points to a communication problem. In this light, the emergence of an illness indicates a functional disturbance which can in principle be avoided to the extent that sufficient risk management is undertaken. Genetic enlightenment (as the deciphering of the 'dark' code) therefore also entails a precise notion of *Mündigkeit* (maturity), which is linked to 'informed decisions' based on the knowledge of one's own genetic risks. In this perspective, the use of genetic diagnosis is not up to individual freedom or personal choice. The will not to know about your genetic make-up or risk profile could be regarded as no will at all: the sign of a deficient or illegitimate will, or even (why not?) the first symptom of a genetic 'disorder'. We might witness a process in which it will be more and more problematic to opt against genetic information and the transmission of this knowledge since this might be seen as an objective witness for lacking moral competence or as an indisputable fact of irrational behaviour (Deftos 1998; Petrila 2001).

Paradoxically, it is exactly the invitation to engage in self-determination and the imperative of a 'genetic responsibility' (Hallowell 1999; Novas and Rose 2000: 21–27) that renders individuals more and more dependent on medico-scientific authorities and their information. The right to health is realized in the form of duty to procure information, and only those who act responsibly draw the correct, i.e. risk-minimizing and forward-oriented, conclusions from this range of information.[3] As a consequence, it is possible to use the experiences with eugenic practices in the past as an instrument to expand moral obligations and duties in the present, as the British Medical Association (BMA) in its report on *Human Genetics: Choice and Responsibility* demonstrates:

> Awareness of abuses practised in the past in the name of 'eugenics' creates an understandable reluctance for health professionals even to think about telling patients who suffer from hereditary conditions that they have special 'duties' to other people or society. The most common 'duty' historically assigned to such patients was that of remaining childless. The BMA maintains, however, that *all patients* have duties of some sort, which may include voluntarily disclosing information to other people who may be affected. Obligations must not be placed on one group – to share information, for example, or limit their reproductive choices – which are not applied to other citizens.
>
> (BMA 1998: 11–12; added emphasis)

The success of this responsibilization strategy depends on a change in the technologies of the self, aiming at 'rational' subjects with 'due foresight' who (wish to) use genetic diagnostics and submit to the resulting decisions or inquire into the specific options which arise. Genetic testing might contribute to constituting a 'homo geneticus' (Gaudillière 1995: 35) who submits to practices of self-control and personal management of the body – which comprises an embodiment of risk technologies that goes well beyond processes of exclusion or mechanisms of repression. The old eugenic programme to achieve 'racial hygiene' which primarily worked by means of coercion and constraint is more and more replaced by the government of genetic risks geared to optimization of human capital in the name of self-determination and individual freedom of choice. This 'genetic responsibility' establishes a new body politic, which calls on us to be as economic as possible with our own body, health or 'quality of life':

> We might say that the political dilemma of eugenics is being solved in the genetic risk society by leaving behind the authoritarian model and replacing it with individualized freedom and responsibility. In the genetic risk society, we may rest assured that most people will make their choices in accordance with the common responsible social rationality.
>
> (Koch 2002: 100)

If this assessment of the link of the concept of genetic risk to a discourse of responsibilization is accurate, then this would entail a fundamentally different meaning being given to eugenics. The notion of the 'purity' of the body of the population which needs to be restored or (re-)created becomes ever more insignificant. As, in principle, everyone is affected by genetic risk and potentially 'ill', current eugenic practices no longer focus on 'purification' of a collective genetic pool, but on 'government' of individual genetic risks. Precisely the construction of genetic risks creates the basis for recoding eugenic practices no longer aimed at specific individuals or identifiable collectives like the criminal subject or the 'feeble-minded', but at each and every single subject. For this reason, today it is probably no longer sufficient to point generally to the risk of eugenics. It might be more accurate to decipher a specific transformation form of eugenics: a eugenics of risk.

Acknowledgements

Many thanks to Monica Greco for 'vital' comments on an earlier version.

Notes

1 For the history of eugenics see Kevles (1985), Schmuhl (1987), Proctor (1988), Adams (1990), Weingart et al. (1992), Kühl (1994); for a bibliographic account of the literature on eugenics, see Beck (1992).

2 However, this does not mean that the (human) genome is a 'social construction', rather the distinction line between the social and technical on the one hand and the natural and biological on the other is itself undergoing a profound transformation. As the historian of science Hans-Jörg Rheinberger remarks:

> [Molecular biology] makes us realize that the result of its scientific conquest is not to supersede, but to change our natural history, that the very essence of our being social is not to supersede, but to alter our natural, that is, in the present context, our genetic condition. We come to realize that the *natural* condition of our genetic makeup might turn into a *social* construct, with the result that the distinction between the "natural" and the "social" no longer makes good sense. We could say as well that the future *social* conditions of man will become based on *natural* constructs. The "natural" and the "social" can no longer be perceived as ontologically different.
>
> (Rheinberger 2000: 29)

3 Hans-Martin Sass, a medical ethical philosopher, therefore calls for an 'ethos of duty' in handling genetic information:

> Leisure time behavior, place of work, or genetic predisposition, or a mixture of all three factors determine the respective individual risks to my health . . . Some can be eliminated, others reduced, or the stage at which they become acute delayed. The patient becomes the partner in preventing or delaying major health risks. The doctor's ethics under the Hippocratic oath, that is characterized by care and outer-determined support, will in future be complemented by a self-determined and self-responsible ethics of the patient and citizen in health-care.
>
> (Sass 1994: 343, translated by TL)

References

Adams, M. (ed.) (1990) *The Wellborn Science: Eugenics in Germany, France, Brazil, and Russia*. New York and Oxford: Oxford University Press.

Beck, C. (1992) *Sozialdarwinismus – Rassenhygiene, Zwangssterilisation und Vernichtung "lebensunwerten" Lebens. Eine Bibliographie zum Umgang mit behinderten Menschen im "Dritten Reich" – und heute*. Bonn: Psychiatrie-Verlag.

Billings, P.R., Kohn, M.A., Cuevas de, M., Beckwith, J., Alper, J.S. and Natowicz, M.R. (1992) 'Discrimination as a consequence of genetic testing', *American Journal of Human Genetics*, 50: 476–482.

Bland, J.S. and Benum, S.H. (1999) *Genetic Nutritioneering. How You Can Modify Inherited Traits and Live a Longer, Healthier Life*. Los Angeles: Keats.

British Medical Association (BMA) (1998) *Human Genetics: Choice and Responsibility*. Oxford: Oxford University Press.

Clark, W.R. (1997) *The New Healers: The Promise and Problems of Molecular Medicine in the Twenty-First Century*. New York and Oxford: Oxford University Press.

Davison, C. (1996) 'Predictive genetics: the cultural implications of supplying probable futures', in T. Marteau and M. Richards (eds) *The Troubled Helix: Social and Psychological Implications of the New Human Genetics*. Cambridge: Cambridge University Press.

Deftos, L.J. (1998) 'The evolving duty to disclose the presence of genetic disease to relatives', *Academic Medicine*, 73: 962–968.

Douglas, M. (1990) 'Risk as a forensic resource', *Daedalus*, 119: 1–16.

Duster, T. (2003) *Backdoor to Eugenics*. New York and London: Routledge.

Foucault, M. (1982) 'The subject and power', in H. Dreyfus and P. Rabinow (eds) *Michel Foucault: Beyond Structuralism and Hermeneutics*. Chicago: University of Chicago Press.

Foucault, M. (1991) 'Governmentality', in G. Burchell, C. Gordon and P. Miller (eds.) *The Foucault Effect*. Hemel Hempstead: Harvester Wheatsheaf.

Gaudillière, J-P. (1995) 'Sequenzieren, Zählen und Vorhersehen. Praktiken einer Genverwaltung', *Tüte*, special issue: Wissen und Macht – Die Krise des Regierens, Tübingen, pp. 34–39.

Hallowell, N. (1999) 'Doing the right thing: genetic risk and responsibility', in P. Conrad and J. Gabe (eds.) *Sociological Perspectives on the New Genetics*. Oxford: Blackwell.

Haraway, D. (1991) *Simians, Cyborgs, and Women: The Reinvention of Nature*. London: Free Association.

Hayes, M.V. (1992) 'On the epistemology of risk – language, logic and social science', *Social Science and Medicine*, 35: 401–407.

Junker, T. and Paul, S. (1999) 'Das Eugenik-Argument in der Diskussion um die Humangenetik: eine kritische Analyse', in E-M. Engels (ed.) *Biologie und Ethik*. Stuttgart: Reclam.

Kay, L.E. (2000) *Who Wrote the Book of Life? A History of the Genetic Code*. Stanford, CA: Stanford University Press.

Keller, E.F. (1992) 'Nature, nurture, and the Human Genome Project', in D.J. Kevles and L. Hood (eds) *The Code of Codes: Scientific and Social Issues in the Human Genome Project*. Cambridge, MA and London: Harvard University Press.

Kenen, R.H. (1996) 'The at-risk health status and technology: a diagnostic invitation and the "gift" of knowing', *Social Science and Medicine*, 42: 1545–1553.

Kevles, D.J. (1985) *In the Name of Eugenics: Genetics and the Uses of Human Heredity*. New York: Alfred A. Knopf.

Kevles, D.J. (1992) 'Out of eugenics: the historical politics of the human genome', in D.J. Kevles and L. Hood (eds) *The Code of Codes: Scientific and Social Issues in the Human Genome Project*. Cambridge, MA and London: Harvard University Press.

Kitcher, P. (1996) *The Lives to Come: The Genetic Revolution and Human Possibilities*. New York and London: Simon & Schuster.

Koch, L. (2002) 'The government of genetic knowledge', in S. Lundin and L. Akesson (eds) *Gene Technology and Economy*. Lund: Nordic Academic.

Koechlin, F. (1996) 'Schön, gesund und ewiger leben', in Frauen gegen Bevölkerungspolitik (ed.) *LebensBilder LebensLügen. Leben und Sterben im Zeitalter der Biomedizin*. Hamburg: Verlag Libertäre Assoziation.

Kühl, S. (1994): *The Nazi Connection: Eugenics, American Racism, and German National Socialism*. Oxford: Oxford University Press.

Latour, B. (1993) *We Have Never Been Modern*. Cambridge, MA: Harvard University Press.

Lemke, T. (1997) *Eine Kritik der politischen Vernunft: Foucaults Analyse der modernen Gouvernementalität*. Berlin: Argument Verlag.

Lemke, T. (2004) Disposition and determinism – genetic diagnosis in risk society. *The Sociological Review*, 52: 550–566.

Low, L., Kind, S. and Wilkie, T. (1998) 'Genetic discrimination in life insurance: empirical evidence from a cross sectional survey of genetic support groups in the United Kingdom', *British Medical Journal*, 317: 1632–1635.

Milunsky, A. (2001) *Your Genetic Destiny: Know your Genes, Secure your Health, Save your Life*. Cambridge, MA: Perseus.

Nassehi, A. (1998) 'Geklonte Götter', *Ästhetik & Kommunikation*, 29: 53–58.

Nelkin, D. and Tancredi, L. (1994) *Dangerous Diagnostics: The Social Power of Biological Information*, 2nd edn. Chicago and London: University of Chicago Press.

Novas, C. and Rose, N. (2000) 'Genetic risk and the birth of the somatic individual', *Economy & Society*, 29: 485–513.

Paul, D.B. (1994) 'Eugenic anxieties, social realities, and political choices', in C.F. Cranor (ed.) *Are Genes Us? The Social Consequences of the New Genetics*. New Brunswick, NJ: Rutgers University Press.

Paul, D.B. (1998) 'Is human genetics disguised eugenics?', in R.F. Weir, S.C. Lawrence and E. Fales (eds) *Genes and Human Self-Knowledge*. Iowa City, IA: University of Iowa Press.

Petersen, A. and Bunton, R. (2002) *The New Genetics and the Public's Health*. London and New York: Routledge.

Petersen, A. and Lupton, D. (1996) *The New Public Health: Health and Self in the Age of Risk*. Thousand Oaks, CA and London: Sage.

Petrila, J. (2001) 'Genetic risk: the new frontier for the duty to warn', *Behavioral Sciences & the Law*, 19: 405–421.

Proctor, R. (1988) *Racial Hygiene: Medicine under the Nazis*. Cambridge, MA: Harvard University Press.

Proctor, R.N. (1992) 'Genomics and eugenics: how fair is the comparison?', in G.J. Annas and S. Elias (eds) *Gene Mapping: Using Law and Ethics as Guides*. New York and Oxford: Oxford University Press.

Propping, P. (1992) 'Was müssen Wissenschaft und Gesellschaft aus der Vergangenheit lernen? Die Zukunft der Humangenetik', in P. Propping and H.

Schrott (eds) *Wissenschaft auf Irrwegen: Biologismus – Rassenhygiene – Eugenik*. Bonn: Bouvier.

Rheinberger, H-J. (2000) 'Beyond nature and culture: modes of reasoning in the age of molecular biology and medicine', in M. Lock, A. Young and A. Cambrosio (eds) *Living and Working with the New Medical Technologies*. Cambridge: Cambridge University Press.

Rose, N. (2000) 'The biology of culpability: pathological identity and crime control in a biological culture'. *Theoretical Criminology*, 4: 5–34.

Rose, N. (2001) 'The politics of life itself', *Theory, Culture and Society*, 18: 1–30.

Rothman, B.K. (1987) *The Tentative Pregnancy: Pre-natal Diagnosis and the Future of Motherhood*. New York: Penguin.

Ruhl, L. (1999) 'Liberal governance and prenatal care: risk and regulation in pregnancy', *Economy and Society*, 28: 95–117.

Sass, H-M. (1994) 'Der Mensch im Zeitalter von genetischer Diagnostik und Manipulation. Kultur, Wissen und Verantwortung', in E.P. Fischer and E. Geißler (eds) *Wieviel Genetik braucht der Mensch? Die alten Träume der Genetiker und ihre heutigen Methoden*. Konstanz: Universitätsverlag Konstanz.

Schmuhl, H-W. (1987) *Rassenhygiene, Nationalsozialismus, Euthanasie. Von der Verhütung zur Vernichtung "lebensunwerten Lebens" 1890–1945*. Göttingen: Vandenhoeck und Ruprecht.

Schumann, M. (1992) 'Vom Sozialdarwinismus zur modernen Reproduktionsmedizin und zur pränatalen Diagnostik – eine kontinuierliche Entwicklung', in A-D. Stein (ed.) *Lebensqualität statt Qualitätskontrolle menschlichen Lebens*. Berlin: Marhold.

Skolbekken, J-A. (1995) 'The risk epidemic in medical journals', *Social Science and Medicine*, 40: 291–305.

Steinberg, D.L. (1996) 'Languages of risk: genetic encryptions of the female body', *Women: a Cultural Review*, 7: 259–270.

Teichler-Zallen, D. (1997) *Does it Run in your Family? A Consumer's Guide to DNA Testing for Genetic Disorders*. New Brunswick, NJ and London: Rutgers University Press.

Thébaud Mondy, A. (1999) 'Genetische Diskriminierung am Arbeitsplatz', *Le Monde Diplomatique*, 14 May: 7.

Weikert, A. (1998) *Genormtes Leben. Bevölkerungspolitik und Eugenik*. Wien: Promedia.

Weingart, P., Kroll, J. and Bayertz, K. (1992) *Rasse, Blut und Gene. Geschichte der Eugenik und Rassenhygiene in Deutschland*. Frankfurt am Main: Suhrkamp.

Weir, L. (1996) 'Recent developments in the government of pregnancy', *Economy & Society*, 25: 372–392.

Wertz, D., Nippert, I. and Wolff, G. (2003) 'Patient and professional responsibilities in genetic counseling', in H-M. Sass and P. Schröder (eds) *Patienten- und Bürgeraufklärung über genetische Risikofaktoren*. Münster: Lit-Verlag.

Winnacker, E-L. (1997) *Das Genom: Möglichkeiten und Grenzen der Genforschung*, 2nd edn. Frankfurt am Main: Eichborn.

Wolff, G. (1990) 'Eugenik und genetische Beratung – Ethische Probleme humangenetischer Diagnostik', *Medizinische Genetik*, 2: 14–20.

Chapter 6

The sociology of the new genetics

Conceptualizing the links between reproduction, gender and bodies

Elizabeth Ettorre

Introduction

Since the late 1980s, we have witnessed a massive proliferation of genetic know-how into many areas of our lives, as Western societies become increasingly dependent upon technological advancements in the new genetics. This development has meant that scientists are able to make biochemical alterations of DNA in cells so as to produce novel, self-reproducing organisms and to think of organisms as disposable (Bowring 2003). More visibly, the new genetics privileged the process of genetic engineering (Minden 1987), viewed as the motor for a new biotechnology (Bud 1993). Through the new genetics, scientists have begun to introduce human choice and design criteria into the construction and combination of genes and paved the way for a 'social-enterepreneurial' approach to genetics (Rose 2003). Biomedical discoveries serve as solutions to a variety of problems found within society, while sophisticated techniques are used as treatments in select cases of individuals, seen as medically and socially deficient (Shakespeare 1995, 1999). Developed from within a scientific culture, whose members have identified traditionally with social progress and humane goals (Foucault 1973), these technologies are not, however, in themselves necessarily benevolent techniques. Nevertheless, the 'tools of post-genomics' have great potential for application to medical research in the coming years (Weatherall 2004).

In this context, the culture of medicine and specifically, the professional practices of physicians with regards to human reproduction have changed dramatically with the swift technological developments, generated by geneticists and microbiologists. The contribution of genetic factors to the entire range of diseases is being recognized, while the public hears that a greater proportion of childhood disease is genetic in origin (Clarke 1997: 5). However, the medical profession's use of genealogical pedigrees to demonstrate that heredity was involved in the aetiology of a particular illness or pathological condition can be traced to the mid-nineteenth century (Resta 1999).

Medical professionals in many countries maintain that most, if not all, women who are pregnant should undergo prenatal diagnosis and be screened for genetic disorders. At the same time, research indicates that men and women in the general population believe that these sorts of techniques can be useful in eliminating a variety of serious diseases (Marteau 1995). As these social trends in the public's perception of genetics materialize, important ethical questions are being raised (Rhodes 1998; Chadwick 2000; Beeson and Doksum 2001). For example, what diseases will be perceived as life threatening? Will 'drug addiction', alcoholism, homosexuality, schizophrenia, severe depression, etc. appear on lists of serious diseases? Will poverty and unemployment be included in this disciplinary process? Will a hierarchy of social diseases be created? If so, who will decide on this hierarchy? Could this hierarchy be used as a basis for social discrimination? Is there an already invisible hierarchy that has developed from the use of prenatal genetic technologies? Most importantly, how do all of these prenatal genetic technologies affect women who are the major recipients of these techniques?

Fashioned by knowledge of the growing impact of biotechnology on medical practice, this chapter highlights some of the key issues that become visible in a sociological analysis of the relationship between reproduction and the new genetics. I use the term 'reproductive genetics' and define it as the utilization of DNA-based technologies in the medical supervision of the reproductive process. In earlier contexts (Ettorre 1999, 2000), I argue that this term is a sociological concept, suggesting that complex social and cultural processes are involved in the organization and use of genetic tests for prenatal diagnosis, already identified as an intricate socio-technological system (Cowan 1994: 35). In feminist contexts, 'reproductive genetics' has been used to demonstrate that it is not possible to treat women and men in the same way with regards reproduction (Mahowald 1994), an issue which has far-reaching ethical implications (Asch and Geller 1996).

My chapter is in two sections. First, I look at the organization of the new genetics through surveillance medicine. Second, I highlight how a mechanistic view of the body is privileged in reproductive genetics. My assumption is that the science of genetics is a part of a disciplinary process, offering a limited view of the human body. This disciplinary process tends to conceal that what may appear as 'flawed genes' is all about bodies' interactions with their surroundings as well as gendered social customs valorized by difference and inflexible definitions of health and illness.

Methodology

The sample

The source of empirical data presented in this chapter is a qualitative study on experts' accounts of the use of prenatal genetic screening in four

European countries: the United Kingdom, Finland, the Netherlands and Greece. This study came from a European consortium of researchers who carried out seven comparative studies in this area. Given that the aim of the experts' study was to review the role of key players influential in public debates in each country, I wanted to find a range of experts who were active in prenatal genetics either clinically or academically. Initially, I hoped to interview at least ten experts in each country and equal numbers of geneticists, clinicians, practitioners, lawyers and/or ethicists, policy-makers, public health officials and researchers. I also decided that besides being known as an 'expert', a prerequisite for inclusion in the study would be fluency in English.

A potential sample of respondents was selected from a list of ten known experts drawn up by collaborating researchers in each country. Experts were known through their publications, work contacts and/or national reputation within relevant networks. A final list for inclusion in the study was drawn up jointly by the author (who would carry out the interviews) and country researchers.

Data collection and analysis

After experts were selected, they were contacted by country researchers and asked whether or not they would be interviewed. With two exceptions, all experts who were selected agreed. With the help of these local researchers, the author set dates when she would be visiting each country as well as arranged times and places for the interviews. Forty-five interviews were included in the study and most were carried out between October 1996 and December 1996. There were seventeen interviews for Finland, ten for Greece, nine for the United Kingdom and nine for the Netherlands. The interviews were conducted in English, tape-recorded and lasted between thirty and ninety minutes: the average was an hour.

It should be noted that although it was possible to reach the desired numbers of interviews in Finland and Greece, this was not possible in the Netherlands and the United Kingdom. Both countries were one short, which was due mainly to the study timetable and budget. All interviews needed to be completed by December 1996 and the researcher had one week's interviewing time in each country. To account for this lack, seven 'unofficial' interviews (i.e. without the use of a tape-recorder) were carried out: four in the Netherlands and three in the United Kingdom. These seven 'unofficial' interviews were mainly with medical students or biomedical researchers with expertise in the area. The data obtained from these 'unofficial' interviews were not used in the data analyses and were perceived by the author as providing background information in specific countries.

Experts were asked their views on genetic testing and screening in prenatal diagnosis. The interview questions revolved around their attitudes on the use of these techniques; their perceptions of the prevailing state of knowledge on legal, medical and ethical aspects; social effects; and policy priorities on local and national levels. All interview data were transcribed and key themes were identified by Word Perfect (Windows) Quick Finder Index. Subsequently, these themes were discussed among collaborating researchers. Excerpts from the experts' interviews will be used in this chapter. I should mention here that some variations of experts' attitudes occurred within specific disciplines (e.g. clinical geneticists disagreed with other clinical geneticists), among disciplines (e.g. differences between clinical geneticists, obstetricians, ethicists, policy-makers) and between countries (e.g. differences between Dutch and UK experts). With regards the last issue, when cross-cultural differences are emphasized, we tend to see less clearly the sorts of interdisciplinary disagreements (i.e. such as those between clinical geneticists and policy-makers, etc.), which are taken for granted in single-country studies (Gilbert and Mulkay 1984; Kerr et al. 1997). The focus in this chapter is mainly on similarities in experts as a group and their attitudes to the use of reproductive genetics. Reporting on these cross-cultural variations has been done in other contexts (Ettorre 1996, 2001; Ettorre et al. 1999).

Surveillance medicine: organising genetics in the community

As a cultural and social system, the medical establishment is a structure of meaning and behavioural norms, attached to particular social relationships and institutional settings (Kleinman 1991). In the light of our topic, it is worthwhile to look at how the cultural meaning of experts and their professional norms are not only shaped by their authoritative claims and relations with those they treat but also practised within specific social settings that change. The assumption, here, is that the current biomedical discourse on the new genetics upholds an observable method of working, facilitating the advancement of sophisticated genetic techniques within a defined group of experts. Thus, how 'genetics work' is organized within biomedicine and what is happening within modern medicine to facilitate the growth of genetics are linked concerns.

Most if not all experts in reproductive genetics have been trained to look for illnesses or diseases in hospitals or clinical settings. Their work has been organized by the dominance of clinical medicine (Foucault 1973) and informed by an 'old' biomedical health care model (Bunton and Burrows 1995). At the same time, the emergence of a newer form of medicine based on surveillance of 'normal' populations has developed. The way in which traditional medical science has established 'the space' for illness (i.e. in hospital or clinic setting) is changing. Health is being redefined in terms that assess levels of functioning and well being in everyday living within social contexts (Tarlov 1996), while the policy challenge focuses a population's attention on preventing disease through public health messages (Blane et al. 1996). Bunton and Burrows (1995: 207) have argued that a new public health has emerged and widens the relevant points of social contacts between professionals and patients into social interactions oriented toward the social body.

In this sense, genetics can be seen to be grounded in this new public health, as it absolves the social structure of responsibility for disease (Wilkinson 1996: 63). One expert referred to the new genetics as a 'public health story' – suggesting that genetics may be a new form of intervention in relation to health and illness:

> Biotechnology and genetics . . . In my opinion, medically speaking, it is a public health story.
>
> (B10 policy-maker)[1]

Atkins and Ahmad (1998: 448) have noted that while the public health message of genetics may emphasize individual decision-making over lifestyles, genetics extends medicine's claims of competence to newer areas of personal and social life, including ideas about appropriate behaviour on the part of patients who are seeking or should be seeking genetic services. Here, one expert believed that the message of genetics should be heard at an early age – becoming a basic component of health prevention and education:

> People should be informed because we can't have relevant discussions about this topic unless people know what they are talking about . . . So I am all for . . . advanced information to the public . . . They are very . . . receptive towards the issue . . . genes, diseased genes . . . if they receive [an] AIDS information package I think that they equally well should receive a genetic information package.
>
> (A3 geneticist)

Additionally for this expert, the appropriate response for a layperson in a public health context was a keen interest in one's 'diseases'. This interest could be elicited also from adolescents – those close to 'a fertile age'. The implication is that adolescents are at a ripe age to digest genetic information and want genetic knowledge, if not services:

> [They should receive] a genetic information package when they are close to the fertile age because . . . there is a keen interest . . . in it. 'What am I?' and 'What diseases are in my family?' . . . So I think that would be the right way to reallocate resources from . . . medical genetics . . . to health education.
>
> (A3 geneticist)

Related to embedding genetics within public health, another expert notes that a general consensus among his colleagues was that appropriate behaviour of an 'aware' 35-year-old pregnant woman was to choose prenatal diagnosis – either amniocentesis or chorionic villus sampling and the inevitability of this choice. However, he believes that constructing a viable public health discourse, enabling one to make this choice, was indeed 'hard work':

> You have this policy through the mass media . . . newspapers . . . the women's magazines . . . that . . . if you are 35 and more you have a great(er) risk to have a baby with Down syndrome or chromosomal abnormalities. We tried very hard actually . . . to convince . . . the patients – the pregnant women – to do amniocentesis or to do CVS for Down syndrome.
>
> (B3 obstetrician)

One expert emphasizes the participatory style and preventative focus of the new public health. She believes that people should be clearly informed of their risks as well as new, available, technologies:

> [There] should be health education to inform people about the risk and the existing techniques and make them available to everybody.
>
> (B9 ethicist)

As the genetics' message is circulated through the new public health, the traditional boundaries between health and illness are breaking down. For example, the paradigm of modern medicine, hospital medicine, has been based on separating those who are 'ill' from those who are 'healthy'. The hospital or the clinic has been the key site for the 'spacialization of illness'. As an institutional setting, the hospital is traditionally the structured space where intervention takes place – where the medical professional observes, manages, treats and diagnoses disease. In this particular social space, illness and disease have a positive visibility with specific signs and symptoms. Medical professionals search for these indications as they focus their medical gaze on the individual.

With the development of the new genetics, a newer paradigm, surveillance medicine (Armstrong 1995) appears more clearly. The site of intervention is the community in contrast to the hospital. It is within this 'new' space of illness – 'the community' – where healthy or unhealthy life styles as well as the combination of genes (i.e. 'faulty' or not), patient carrier status and risk factors are identified.

Confirming the community as a viable site for intervention, one expert spoke about setting up 'a gene shop' and how this would be an important way of generating interest and public awareness:

> I am involved in . . . running the gene shop .... to increase the level of public awareness and . . . knowledge . . . [So] that when somebody . . . says, 'Would

you like a triple test?', they thought that through . . . They know . . . those that said, 'Yes' have said 'Yes' because they understand why they say 'Yes' a bit more . . . It means to have anything to do with genetics ventilated in the widest possible way . . . making knowledge freely available.

(D3 clinical geneticist)

In this movement from hospital to surveillance medicine, there is a shift in modern medical culture from looking at subjective signs and symptoms that sufferers, consumers, patients, etc. experience when they feel sick to performing objective tests in the community. One expert illustrates this point vividly when he discusses the development of a new technology, analysis of foetal cells. He describes how this is being developed with the explicit intention of screening large groups of low-risk women, previously outside of the scope of reproductive genetics. Stating that this needs to be highly organized in order to be effective, he implies that if analysis of foetal cells becomes routinized, there will no longer be a need for maternal serum screening, CVS or amniocentesis – the latter described as 'the gold standard' in prenatal diagnosis (Kuller and Laifer 1995). A DNA test on foetal cells in the mother's blood is all that would be done – 'no risk', 'no fuss'. But, technically, this is not 'yet' possible. This expert envisages that most if not all pregnancies will come under the domain of large-scale DNA-based prenatal screening programmes. If analysis of foetal cells materialized, this technology could spearhead the mass use of genetic tests in the community:

[I] am talking about the possibilities of large group screening of low-risk pregnancies for chromosomal abnormalities, by looking at foetal cells in maternal circulation . . . At the moment . . . it doesn't work as a test to be performed on a large scale . . . If there is a real good programme available for large-scale detection . . . it's only possible to do it well, if you have a very high level of organization.

(C4 clinical geneticist)

Another expert confirmed the possible proliferation of foetal cell analysis in the community and described this as 'magnificent'.

It would be magnificent if there were a movement towards that . . . in the future. Because if it will be a diagnostic procedure, then it will be magnificent . . . you don't need amniocentesis or CVS any more . . . if it is a diagnostic procedure . . . It will be too easy for people to do that . . . Now they . . . have to think about it. What is more important – having an abortion after amniocentesis or the child with Down syndrome . . . ? But if you are only to take some blood from your arm and you know the result . . . it will be too easy for them to have their blood examined and then they know I will get a child with Down syndrome and now, do I want an abortion for it?

(C6 gynaecologist)

This suggests that a shift from looking at subjective signs and symptoms of individuals to objective tests with most if not all pregnant women in the community, accelerates the proliferation of these technologies into previously untouched social spaces.

While reproductive genetics is being increasingly shaped by strategies of surveillance medicine, it is a belief among some physicians that the health of a community will be ensured only if the whole of the population comes within the range of genetic surveillance. Within this paradigm, there could arise a danger that genetic prediction will become linked, if not equated with disease prevention. Perhaps this link is already being established, as one expert suggests:

> People are now interested to ask questions about prenatal diseases. They are interested in knowing what kind of child they will have . . . because abortion is possible . . . If there is a psychological or any other problem illness . . . abortion is possible . . . People know that there is a system . . . a way to determine the health of the child.
>
> (B10 policy-maker)

The scientific scope for the development of genetic technologies may appear endless as techniques, the range of knowledge and knowledge interests, and work organization within surveillance medicine continue to grow. Genetic technologies embody complex social relationships and experts involved in these relationships are integral to surveillance medicine, the cultural configuration in which reproductive genetics is currently being reproduced.

Reclaiming the genetics agenda: containing diversity and shaping bodies

Social scientists who engage with this genetic discourse must be aware of how surveillance medicine encourages the genetics agenda in society. In this context, Lippman (1992) is concerned about geneticization and asks what if we changed genetic metaphors and for example, see a gene map as no more than an organogram (i.e. the grand bureaucratic design of an organization – fixed and orderly). She asks further, 'Do we really want to invest major human or economic resources in the development of an organogram?' Her main aim in asking these questions is to call for a reclaiming of the genetic agenda by a thorough exposure of the genetic colonization of health and illness in and through the narrative of contemporary genetics.

While it has been argued that human genetics is the science of difference (Murray and Livny 1995), genetics is a part of a collective process – science – in which scientists attempt to legitimize the 'principle of dominance' (Haraway 1991) or what has been called the 'episteme of domination' (Benhabib 1990). This 'episteme of domination' is characterized by the knowledge seeker's (i.e. scientist's, medical professional's, etc.) quest for control as well as the imposition of a certain level of homogeneity on the world. As scientists seek for understanding of the human genome through concept building and utilization of genetic technologies, they appear as wanting to impose 'sameness' or homogeneity on society. On the other hand, as Hartouni suggests:

> Sameness, repetition, and replication . . . are not the issue, at least not in the terms in which they have been presented as such. The issue, rather, is how to conventionalise and contain diversity and (the proliferation of) difference(s) or how to render diversity and difference socially legible, and that is what geneticizing both would seem in the end, at least ostensibly to accomplish.
>
> (Hartouni 1997: 119)

In the process of reclaiming the genetics agenda, we as social scientists need to contextualize the human body as a politically inscribed entity, its biology and pedigree shaped by histories/herstories and practices of containment and control as well as difference. In our analysis, we need to place the body at the core of political struggles (Turner 1996: 67). Bodies need to be seen as sites where the knowledge of genes, foetuses, reproductive functions and the universalizing system of surveillance medicine converge and not as gender neutral, non-determinate systems. One difficulty is that this work needs to be done with the explicit intention of demonstrating how notions of 'genes in bodies', the paradigm about healthy and diseased genes, and ideas about appropriate kinds and levels of reproductive performances are culturally dependent 'embodied processes'. Thus, this work is about the need for a resurrection of the body in our work and the breathing of 'epistemological' life back into our neglected frames. Our work is about the affirmation of corporeality – making the distinct claim that the body exists very centrally in the genetics discourse. To make this claim is to understand more fully why specific genetic metaphors have been needed not only as rhetorical tools but also as active agents in forming a genetic 'moral order' which is dispersed in a multiplicity of ways with far-reaching effects.

For example, the circulation of symbols, images and myths about genes 'in bodies' permeate the fabric of contemporary society (Wark 2002). Used regularly, metaphors signal the proliferation of genetic knowledge and technologies into our everyday life. Nelkin and Lindee (1995: 6) contend that there are three related themes that underlie the metaphors geneticists and other biologists use to describe work on the human genome. These include the characterization of the gene as the essence of identity; a promise that genetic research will enhance prediction of human behaviour and health; and an image of the genome as a text that will define the natural order. They envisage the gene as a cultural icon, exalted above everything else in human nature – a type of omnipotent signifier. In related contexts, Hubbard and

Wald (1993) attempt to explode the gene myth and suggest that the search for the human genome can be likened to the quest for the Holy Grail – a quest for the sacred object of Western civilization which ended up to be a prolonged pursuit carried out mainly by privileged men (i.e. knights) during the Middle Ages. Other scholars (Rosner and Johnson 1995: 104), familiar with these kinds of genetic metaphors, suggest that, whether living (i.e. stories) or dead (i.e. inanimate objects), these metaphors 'invariably cast the scientist as the one who dominates and exploits the Other'.

Also, genetic metaphors have in common the idea that genes can be precisely spatialized – captured in a gaze, charted or measured. On the one hand, every scientist knows genes are located in bodies. On the other hand, in order to hallow genes and empower technology, scientists need metaphors, protecting the primacy of the gene – not the body. As Gottweis (1997: 57) exclaims, 'We are our genes. Eureka!' In this logic, scientists uphold the view that genes – not bodies – determine human social behaviour. They believe that genes, active in various combinations rather than bodies, inscribed by culture, are fundamental in explaining social performance. As biology and genetics are pushed into the foreground of social consciousness, culture takes a back seat, if any at all. In effect, this process obliterates the fact that bodies are marked by categories of difference (i.e. gender, race and disability). It establishes the body as 'but an epiphenomenon of its genes' (Gilbert 1997: 40). In the sphere of reproductive genetics, the bodies of pregnant women and disabled people fall outside of the paradigm of health or well-being, as the former bodies are being invaded while the latter, are eliminated. Medical technology drives this process, whether living bodies are invaded or potential bodies eliminated.

Besides metaphors, powerful genetic concepts are used in reproductive genetics to help circulate a genetic moral order. For example, concepts such as 'risk', 'affected offspring', 'viability', 'defective genes', 'carrier status', etc. are mobilized by experts to mark 'harmony' or 'disharmony' in the progression of women's reproductive process and ultimately, between herself as a pregnant woman and her foetus.

Contextualizing the links: genetics, gender and female bodies

In recent work (Ettorre 2000, 2002), I contend that social scientists should view the whole of the genetics discourse including reproductive genetics, as raising important issues around discourses on the body. Indeed, an understanding of the body is important for a sophisticated history of medical knowledge (Turner 1992). As the body focused on in genetics is more often than not a female body, one assumes that these technologies tend to be directed more towards women's bodies than men's bodies. Thus, at the meeting point between surveillance medicine and the new genetics is a focus on the body – a body interacting within the community and a body as the specific site for gathering genetic material. It is 'within' this physical body that scientists are able to see the structure of the material of genes – DNA. But, this physical body, the original site for foetal (Newman 1996) and/or genetic investigations, is shaped by gender. The scientific gaze in the field of genetics tends to be increasingly on the physical body – a pregnant body – a gendered, female body. In turn, reproductive limits are practised on this gendered body through a feminized regime of reproductive asceticism and involvement in a discourse on shame (Ettorre 2000).

The fact that pregnant women are somehow captured in discourses on the body is not by chance. Through the current developments in genetics, members of the public as well as the medical profession are required to consider the desire for healthy descendants (or what I have referred to as those with 'good' genetic capital). One could predict that as genetic screening increases, pregnant women's bodies will be the major recipients of these screening programmes. This will be related to the priority society places on women's reproductive role as well as the increasing management of the pregnant body by the medical profession – what has been traditionally called 'medicalization'. While this research area has been already documented (Graham and Oakley 1986), we should not lose sight of the fact that medicalization is alive and well in reproductive genetics (Ettorre 1999).

From the above, we have seen that the concepts and ideas utilized in reproductive genetics appear to exert more restraint and impose more limitations on women's than men's bodies. In this context, the construction of the body has been the effect of endless circulation of power and knowledge (Bordo 1993: 21). This body, as gendered, raced, aged and marked by anatomical, cerebral or physiological difference or damage, provides the focus for regulatory techniques which are practised on the individual, particularly a pregnant woman, as a living body. These regulatory techniques are continually being played out through reproductive genetics and reproductive health care. The external problem of regulating a consuming body and the internal problem of exerting self-restraint on a reproducing body merge with the result that shame, as an experience bound by gender, performs a regulatory function. The morality of the body during pregnancy demands order or genetic harmony. For women, 'fit or viable foetuses' means they have fit bodies and they can share in this harmony. While unfit foetuses may imply states of disharmony and potential ill-health, the self-restraint practised through their reproductive asceticism comes to be seen as a failure in the eyes of these 'bad reproducers'.

Conclusion

This chapter reported on findings from an empirical study of European experts. We have seen how genetics is mobilized through surveillance medicine and how a mechanistic view of the body is privileged in reproductive genetics. We also saw how reproductive genetics has particular effects on bodies, specifically women's bodies. As sociologists we have the important task of uncovering some of the unintended consequences of the new genetics. Reproductive genetics embodies complex gendered relationships and processes. Thus, social scientists should fully investigate and explore these relationships and processes. Alongside medical colleagues, they need to become key players or producers of ideas in a society in which genetic knowledge is being privileged on a steady basis. To challenge the privileging of genetic knowledge will not be an easy task, but they should embrace this challenge with the power and tools of the social sciences.

Note

1 All interviews are numbered in chronological order. A stands for Finland, B for Greece, C for the Netherlands and D for the United Kingdom. D1 indicates the first interview carried out in the United Kingdom.

References

Armstrong, D. (1995) 'The rise of surveillance medicine', *Sociology of Health and Illness*, 17(3): 393–404.

Asch, A. and Geller, G. (1996) 'Feminism, bioethics and genetics', in S. Wolfe (ed.) *Feminism and Bioethics: Beyond Reproduction.* Oxford: Oxford University Press.

Atkins, K. and Ahmad, W. (1998) 'Genetic screening and haemoglobinopathies: ethics, politics and practice', *Social Science and Medicine*, 46(3): 445–458.

Beeson, D. and Doksum, T. (2001) 'Family values and resistance to genetic testing', in B. Hoffmaster (ed.) *Bioethics in Social Context.* Philadelphia, PA: Temple University Press.

Benhabib, S. (1990) 'Epistemologies of postmodernism: a rejoinder to Jean Francois Lyotard', in L.J. Nicholson (ed.) *Feminism/Postmodernism.* London: Routledge.

Blane, D., Brunner, E. and Wilkinson, R. (1996) 'The evolution of public health policy: an anglocentric view of the last fifty years', in D. Blane, E. Brunner and R. Wilkinson (eds.) *Health and Social Organization: Towards a Health Policy for the Twenty-first Century.* London: Routledge.

Bordo, S. (1993) *Unbearable Weight: Feminism, Western Culture and the Body.* Berkeley, CA: University of California Press.

Bowring, F. (2003) *Science Seeds and Cyborgs: Biotechnology and the Appropriation of Life.* London: Verso.

Bud, R. (1993) *The Uses of Life: A History of Biotechnology.* Cambridge: Cambridge University Press.

Bunton, R. and Burrows, R. (1995) 'Consumption and health in the "epidemiological" clinic of late modern medicine', in R. Bunton, S. Nettleton and R. Burrows (eds) *The Sociology of Health Promotion.* London: Routledge.

Chadwick, R. (2000) 'Ethical issues in psychiatric care: geneticisation and community care', *Act Psychiatrica Scandinavica*, 101(Supplement 399): 35–39.

Clarke, A. (1997) 'Introduction', in A. Clarke and E. Parsons (eds) *Culture, Kinship and Genes: Towards Cross-cultural Genetics*. London: Macmillan.

Cowan, R.S. (1994) 'Women's roles in the history of amniocentesis and chorionic villi sampling', in K. Rothenberg and E.J. Thomson (eds) *Women and Prenatal Testing: Facing the Challenges of Genetic Testing*. Columbus, OH: Ohio State University Press.

Ettorre, E. (1996) *The New Genetics Discourse in Finland: Exploring Experts' Views Within Surveillance Medicine*. Helsinki: Suomen Kuntaliitto (Association of Finnish Metropolitan Authorities)

Ettorre, E. (1999) 'Experts as genetic storytellers: exploring key issues', *Sociology of Health and Illness*, 21(5): 539–559.

Ettorre, E. (2000) 'Reproductive genetics, gender and disability: "Please doctor, may I have a normal baby?"', *Sociology*, 34(3): 403–420.

Ettorre, E. (ed.) (2001) *Before Birth*. London: Ashgate.

Ettorre, E. (2002) *Reproductive Genetics, Gender and the Body*. London: Routledge.

Ettorre, E., Hemminki, E., Aro, A, Dragonas, T., Adams, E., Van de Hueval, W., Tymstra, T. and Alderson, P. (1999) *Final Report of the European Union Project on the Development of Prenatal Screening in Europe: The Past, the Present and the Future*. Helsinki: University of Helsinki.

Foucault, M. (1973) *The Birth of the Clinic*. London: Tavistock.

Gilbert, S.F. (1997) 'Bodies of knowledge: biology and the intercultural university', in P. Taylor, S. Halfron and P. Edwards (eds) *Changing Life: Genomes, Ecologies, Bodies and Commodities*. Minneapolis, MN: University of Minnesota Press.

Gilbert, N. and Mulkay M. (1984) *Opening Pandora's Box: A Sociological Analysis of Scientist's Discourse*. Cambridge: Cambridge University Press.

Gottweis, H. (1997) 'Genetic engineering, discourses of deficiency and the new politics of population', in P. Taylor, S. Halfron and P. Edwards (eds) *Changing Life: Genomes, Ecologies, Bodies and Commodities*. Minneapolis, MN: University of Minnesota Press.

Graham, H. and Oakley, A. (1986) 'Competing ideologies of reproduction: medical and maternal perspectives on pregnancy', in C. Currer and M. Stacey (eds) *Concepts of Health, Illness and Disease*. Leamington Spa: Berg.

Haraway, D. (1991) *Simians, Cyborgs and Women*. London and New York: Routledge.

Hartouni, V. (1997) *Cultural Conceptions on Reproductive Technologies and the Remaking of Life*. Minneapolis, MN: University of Minnesota Press.

Hubbard, R. and Wald, E. (1993) *Exploding the Gene Myth*. Boston, MA: Beacon Press.

Kerr, A., Cunningham-Burley, S. and Amos, A. (1997) 'The new genetics: professionals' discursive boundaries', *Sociological Review*, 45(2): 297–303.

Kleinman, A. (1991) 'Concepts and a model for the comparison of medical systems as cultural systems', in C. Currer and M. Stacey (eds) *Concepts of Health, Illness and Disease*, 2nd edn. Oxford: Berg.

Kuller, J.A. and Laifer, S.A. (1995) 'Contemporary approaches to prenatal diagnosis', *American Family Physician*, 52(8): 2277–2283.

Lippman, A. (1992) 'Led (astray) by genetic maps: the cartography of the human genome and health care', *Social Science and Medicine*, 35(12): 1469–1476.

Mahowald, M.B. (1994) 'Reproductive genetics and gender justice', in K. Rothenberg and E.J. Thomson (eds) *Women and Prenatal Testing: Facing the Challenges of Genetic Testing*. Columbus, OH: Ohio State University Press.

Marteau, T.M. (1995) 'Towards informed decisions about prenatal testing: a review', *Prenatal Diagnosis*, 15: 1215–1226.

Minden, S. (1987) 'Patriarchal designs: the genetic engineering of human embryos', in P. Spallone and D.L. Steinberg (eds) *Made to Order: The Myth of Reproductive and Genetic Engineering*. Oxford: Pergamon Press.

Murray, T.H. and Livny, E. (1995) 'The Human Genome Project: ethical and social implications', *Bulletin of the Medical Library Association*, 83(1): 14–21.

Nelkin, D. and Lindee, S. (1995) *The DNA Mystiques: The Gene as a Cultural Icon*. New York: W.H. Freeman.

Newman, K. (1996) *Fetal Positions: Individualism, Science and Visuality*. Stanford, CA: Stanford University Press.

Resta, R. (1999) 'A brief history of the pedigree in human genetics', in R.A. Peel (ed.) *Human Pedigree Studies*. London: Galton Institute.

Rhodes, R. (1998) 'Genetic links, family ties, and social bonds: rights and responsibilities in the face of genetic knowledge', *Journal of Medicine and Philosophy*, 23(1): 10–30.

Rose, H. (2003) 'An ethical dilemma: the rise and fall of UmanGenomics – the model biotech company?', *Nature*, 425: 123–124.

Rosner, M. and Johnson, T.R. (1995) 'Telling stories: metaphors of the Human Genome Project', *Hypatia*, 10(4): 104–129.

Shakespeare, T. (1995) 'Back to the future? New genetics and disabled people', *Critical Social Policy*, 15: 22–35.

Shakespeare, T. (1999) 'Losing the plot? Medical and activist discourses of contemporary genetics and disability', *Sociology of Health and Illness*, 21(5): 669–688.

Tarlov, A.R. (1996) 'Social determinants of health: the sociobiological translation', in D. Blane, E. Brunner and R. Wilkinson (eds) *Health and Social Organization: Towards a Health Policy for the Twenty-first Century*. London: Routledge.

Turner, B. (1992) *Regulating Bodies: Essays in Medical Sociology*. London: Routledge.

Turner, B. (1996) *The Body and Society*. London: Sage.

Wark, M. (2002) 'Codework: from cyberspace to biospace, from Neuromancer to Gattaca', in J. Armitage and J. Roberts (eds) *Living with Cyberspace: Technology and Society in the 21st Century*. London: Continuum.

Weatherall, D.J. (2004) 'Genetics and the future of medicine', in M. Keynes, A.W.F. Edwards and R. Peel (eds) *A Century of Mendelism in Human Genetics*. London: CRC Press.

Wilkinson, R.G. (1996) *Unhealthy Societies: The Afflictions of Inequality*. London: Routledge.

Chapter 7

Whose right to choose?

The new genetics, prenatal testing and people with learning difficulties

Linda Ward

Introduction

In the summer of 1998, Inclusion International (formerly, ILSMH – the International League of Societies for people with Mental Handicap) held a conference in The Hague. A key symposium focused on the implications of the new genetics for people with learning difficulties. The title – 'To be or not to be?' – was emotive. But it reflected the unease felt by some disabled people and their families about developments in genetic technology and prenatal diagnosis, and their implications.

Advances in genetic knowledge and the huge proliferation of prenatal tests, have mostly *not* (yet) led to therapy, treatment or 'cure' for a foetus detected as having an impairment. The anticipated outcome of a positive prenatal test for impairment remains abortion. Hardly surprising, then, that many in the disability community, and their supporters, are deeply concerned that societal acceptance, even welcoming, of increased genetic testing signals powerful messages about the value placed on disabled people's lives – and even their fundamental right 'to be'.

There are 'many interests' at work in developments in genetic technology (Rioux 2001). At the forefront of these have been the biochemists and geneticists for whom the consequences of plotting the human genome are of enormous scientific, medical (and commercial) consequence. Media coverage of the endeavour to map the human genome, and reports of 'discoveries' and developments in related technologies, have been largely positive about their implications for science, for society, and for people with inherited, or long-term, ultimately life-threatening conditions, like sickle-cell anaemia, Huntington's disease or cystic fibrosis.

The darker side of this apparently positive picture has received much less exposure. This is due, in part, to the profound 'silences in the public discourse' in this area (Press 2000): that is, the lack of explicit, public, acknowledgement that the outcome of increased prenatal screening and testing is an increase in abortion on the grounds of foetal impairment. This silence has facilitated the rapid growth and routinization of prenatal testing, without concurrent public debate on the two issues most centrally involved: disability and abortion. Fundamental issues and assumptions implicit in routine practice are rarely surfaced and reviewed. Hence this chapter which seeks to explore some critical questions in this area, in particular in relation to people with learning (intellectual) disabilities and their families. For example:

- What are the wider implications of the increasing preoccupation with the prevention of impairment through prenatal diagnosis?
- What do current policies and practices around prenatal testing (followed by selective abortion) signal about societal acceptance of diversity, difference and disabled people?
- How do we reconcile an increased, overt, emphasis on 'parental choice' in this area (that is, whether to proceed with, or terminate, an affected pregnancy) with the knowledge that prenatal genetic testing programmes are instituted on an assumption of cost-effectiveness? (Prenatal testing programmes may be presented as an extension of parental choice, but that 'choice' needs to operate predominantly in favour of the termination of an affected pregnancy for programmes to operate cost-effectively.)

The views and voices of people with learning disabilities have not been prominent in public debate on these issues, for reasons which are explored in more detail later (these include their marginal position in relation to the disability movement generally; difficulties with literacy; problems in accessing, and understanding, complex and abstract debate of this kind). This chapter begins, therefore, by reviewing some of the critical arguments put forward by people *with physical impairments* on the implications of the new genetics and developments in prenatal testing for disabled people and disability rights generally. Only then does it move on to consider the particular (and hitherto ignored) issues affecting people with learning disabilities. It describes an innovative initiative aimed at making information on the subject accessible to them, soliciting their views on policies and practice in this area, and subsequently negotiating the difficulties inherent in developing a strategy for making available accessible information on the issue to people with learning disabilities more widely.

The chapter concludes with a review of the issues and assumptions demanding further public attention in a society now officially committed (via the United Kingdom Disability Discrimination Act 1995 and Disability Rights Commissions) to combating discrimination against disabled people and promoting their equal rights.

Prenatal diagnosis: a disability rights critique

Jenny Morris's classic work, *Pride against Prejudice: Transforming Attitudes to Disability* (Morris 1991), provides one of the earliest reviews in the United Kingdom of the issues posed by developments in genetic technology and prenatal diagnosis for disabled people. Her chapter, 'The chance of life', not only explores the issues surrounding prenatal testing and abortion, from a disability rights perspective, but also explicitly exposes, and grapples with, the tensions between a (feminist) commitment to parental choice ('a woman's right to choose' when and whether to continue a pregnancy) and the concerns of the disability movement about the societal values implicit in the assumption that increased prenatal testing to detect impairment, followed by abortion of affected foetuses, is clearly desirable.

Morris's analysis illuminates some critical points within these problematic areas: the assumption that the presence of an impairment makes the birth of a foetus automatically unwelcome; legal support for that position within UK legislation (in cases where the foetus is thought to have a serious impairment, there is no time limit for the termination of that pregnancy, while for other pregnancies the time limit is 24 weeks); an assumption about the poor quality of life inevitable for a disabled child and its family (which fails to take account of the societal circumstances which contribute to these stresses); the societal constraints within which women 'choose' not to have a disabled child (for example, inadequate services and support and discrimination against disabled people); lack of protection for the rights of the unborn child with an impairment; and the cost–benefit analyses which judge the birth of disabled children an unnecessary and unwelcome burden in economic terms. This analysis is enhanced by its context. The preceding chapter explores in detail the idea that the lives of disabled people are 'lives not worth living', reminding the reader of other social policies of recent times, which have similarly devalued and discounted the lives of disabled people – most notably the eugenics movement in the early part of the twentieth century, national policies of compulsory sterilization (cf. Herbert 1997) and the Nazi 'euthanasia' programme under which an estimated one hundred thousand disabled people were killed by the Third Reich (Sutherland 1981).

The potentially conflicting tensions between the two apparent goals of prenatal testing – increasing parental choice and the prevention of impairment – are explored in more detail by Ruth Bailey (1996). Bailey looks specifically at the implications of prenatal testing for disabled people, in the light of advances in genetic knowledge, with a particular focus on what this means for women.

Non-disabled feminists have, on the whole, welcomed prenatal testing as another means by which women can gain control over their own reproduction, though some feminist writers (e.g. Rothman 1984) have made clear the price paid for that 'choice' or control (for example, having to decide whether to undergo tests; awaiting results; subsequent decision-making about continuing a pregnancy or electing for abortion). But for many disabled women (including disabled feminists) the feminist defence of selective abortion in the case of suspected impairment (on the grounds of 'a woman's right to choose') has raised sharp questions about the prejudicial assumptions implicit here and the differential values ascribed to the lives of foetuses with, and without, a detectable impairment.

Bailey explores the assumptions at the heart of prenatal testing: in the medical and scientific context in which it takes place, and in the social policies and legislative framework surrounding it. The emphasis throughout all these is on impairment prevention: 'Prenatal testing is rarely done so that a condition can be treated in either the mother or the foetus' (Bailey 1996: 145); the presumption is that prenatal testing followed by selective abortion is right, even ethical, because it can prevent suffering, through the termination of the impaired pregnancy. There has, however, been no explicit debate within the medical profession of what degrees or types of impairment lead to such a level of suffering that offering an abortion must be justified, and there is no official consensus on this issue.

Bailey's work poses a number of key questions relevant to this chapter. First, why is Down syndrome one of the two most common conditions for which prenatal testing is offered, given that people with Down syndrome rarely suffer physical pain or distress as a direct result of their primary impairment (though they may well suffer from other conditions in addition) and it is arguable whether the impairment could be described as 'serious' (as defined by the Human Fertilisation and Embryology Act 1990)? Is prenatal testing for Down syndrome more about preventing the 'suffering' (social or psychological) of others (for example, parents) than of the individual directly affected?

Second, how do the attitudes of medical professionals towards disability and impairment impact on the operation of prenatal testing programmes? If 'the case for prenatal testing is self evident and largely unproblematic' for the medical profession generally (Bailey 1996: 150) such attitudes are likely to impact on women's views of impairment and disability, their attitudes towards selective abortion in particular, and their likelihood of exercising choice in favour of termination of an affected pregnancy. Indeed, Bailey (1996: 152) argues that the increased availability of prenatal testing has 'institutionalised the fear of impairment', increasing the value attached to non-disabled children (cf. Alderson 2001).

Third, the scientific context of prenatal testing also plays a critical role. 'Science' is traditionally portrayed as 'value free' in its presentation of such issues, but Bailey pinpoints three causes for concern in relation to the development of genetic research: the representation of genetic impairment as a definitive category; the assumption that impairment is a wholly negative experience; the ensuing risk that the political and medical agenda in this area is set by 'what science has now enabled us to do' (Bailey 1996: 155), for example, in terms of what tests are available (cf. Clarke 1993).

Fourth, how does the state's *implicit* interest in prenatal diagnosis (particularly its economic interests in preventing the birth of children with impairments) impact upon the *explicit* aims of prenatal diagnosis, which are said to be about affording prospective parents the chance to make informed choices? The 'effectiveness' of prenatal diagnosis is determined by health economists, via cost–benefit analyses which set the resources invested in screening against the savings that result; that is the savings to the state of the costs of supporting a disabled child. (For example, if fewer than 50 per cent of parents opted for abortion when a foetus was diagnosed with a disorder, that programme would be deemed 'a failure': Institute of Medicine 1994). Such analyses make clear (though not explicit) that the state's interest in prenatal testing is not about women making *any* informed choice but about making a *particular* choice, namely to have an abortion.

A key concern for Bailey and other disabled commentators has been the domination of the discourse in this area by scientists, the medical profession and health economists – and the minimal space afforded to the perspectives of the disability community, arguably key stakeholders in this debate. But since the early 1990s significant contributions have been made to the debate by disabled people in the United Kingdom (e.g. Fletcher 1997, 1999, 2000, 2001; All Party Parliamentary Disablement Group 1999), in Europe (Disabled Peoples' International 1998) and in North America (Finger 1991; Kaplan and other contributors to Rothenberg and Thomson 1994; Saxton 2000). (See also special issue on disability and bioethics, *Disability Tribune* newsletter, February 2000.)

Of particular significance, perhaps, for this chapter have been the contributions by Tom Shakespeare, a British disabled academic with achondroplasia (restricted growth) not only through his prolific writings in academic journals and the popular and quality press, but also on television (see, for example, *Ivy's Genes*, Isis Productions, Channel 4, 1995) and through regular contributions to events organized by the disability community (Shakespeare 1998) and elsewhere (including, for example, at the Labour Party conference in England, September 2000: Shakespeare 2000). Shakespeare's experience demonstrates painfully well the diversity of opinion, difficulties and dilemmas for disabled people and their (prospective) families in relation to developments in genetic technology, not least the tension between the extension of parental choice on the one hand and the prevention of impairment on the other. At the Labour Party conference fringe meeting, for example, Shakespeare was accused of 'removing hope' from fellow disabled people with inherited, life-threatening conditions like cystic fibrosis, who live in anticipation of genetic therapies and cures for their conditions because of his sceptical critique of genetic developments (Shakespeare 2000); yet at the same time some (but by no means all) fellow disability activists have been sharp in their criticism of him, for saying that he could understand that some prospective parents might want genetic screening to avoid the birth of a very severely disabled child (*Disability Now*, May 2000).

The single, most comprehensive, yet accessible, resource on these complex issues on either side of the Atlantic, is *Prenatal Testing and*

Rights Disability (Parens and Asch 2000a). The edited collection is the product of a two-year project based in New York, which brought together disabled people, parents with disabled children and experts in disability studies, medical genetics, genetic counselling, medicine, law, the humanities and social sciences. The resulting volume provides detailed coverage of the multiplicity of issues and perspectives within the complex area of prenatal diagnosis and disability rights, with a final section 'Making policies, delivering services', addressing the implications for policy and practice. The book offers no easy answers to the multiple dilemmas in this field; significantly, the group itself was unable to reach consensus on a number of issues. It does, however surface many of the hidden assumptions – and tensions – currently implicit in societal attitudes to, and provision of, prenatal testing and selective abortion, and provides much material relevant to three questions critical to the focus of this chapter.

Is prenatal testing just a natural extension of good prenatal care?

Prenatal screening is subsumed under the rubric of routine prenatal care only by virtue of the fact that an assumption of abortion in the case of a suspected impairment is not talked about (Press 2000: 221). This may be deliberate. Press (2000: 221) notes that 'health care providers . . . were often quite open about the fact that the link between abortion and prenatal screening was intentionally avoided' in public discussion. Indeed, she points out that

> a truly open approach to the centrality of abortion to prenatal screening is found almost exclusively in the cost benefit analysis done on MSAFP [Maternal Serum Alpha Feta Protein screening – for neural tube defects] and other prenatal screening.
>
> (Press 2000)

If society were truly serious about reducing impairment, other health promotion strategies (less directly under the influence of the medical profession and scientists) might be equally viable, and arguably more valuable. Bailey, for example, describes the reluctance of the United Kingdom government to insist on the forcible addition of folic acid to bread as the surest way of ensuring all women got sufficient quantities, with a possible reduction thereby of the incidence of neural tube defects by 75%. Such a stance conflicted with the government's commitment to the deregulation of industry (Bailey 1996). Similarly, Williams (1997) shows that a serious commitment to reducing impairments would involve close attention to the social and environmental factors so commonly involved.

Does prenatal testing really offer parents 'the right to choose'?

Given the pressure on women both to undergo tests, and to opt for an abortion in the event of a detected impairment (cf. Dodds 1997), the evidence suggests that the choices available are highly circumscribed. Jennings (2000) makes a powerful argument *against* the value neutrality of genetic technology and indeed, the lack of neutrality of information offered to prospective parents via genetic counselling also: 'The counselling may be neutral as regards the personal beliefs of the counsellor, but it cannot be neutral as regards the very context of genetic technology itself' (Jennings 2000: 136). Dorothy Wertz's questionnaire surveys of genetics professionals, including geneticists and genetic counsellors in the United States and elsewhere, provide support for this view. While 'most genetic services providers said they would be non directive in counselling about most conditions', they were, in fact, much more likely to abort for these conditions than primary care physicians (Wertz 2000: 278). Hence, the need for changes in the delivery of prenatal genetic information to take account of the concerns of the disability community (Bieseker and Hamby 2000).

What messages does prenatal testing, followed by selective abortion of foetuses with an impairment, send to the rest of society about the value placed on its disabled citizens?

This is the so-called 'expressivity' argument: the argument that the assumptions implicit in accepted practice regarding the abortion of foetuses with detected impairments, send out clear (and negative) signals about the value society places on its disabled members (Parens and Asch 2000b). Given that much of the disadvantage experienced by disabled people in our society is *socially* rather than (exclusively) *genetically* created, what are the implications of prenatal testing programmes for an 'impairment trait' (Morris 1996)? Many contributors to Parens and Asch's volume take the view that impairment (or disability) is a 'neutral' trait in itself, and that tests for it, followed by selective abortion, are as morally unacceptable as testing for similarly 'neutral' traits, like race or gender. Disabled commentators note, in addition, the tendency for the medical community to 'take the part for the whole'. 'When we present the diagnosis of a genetic disease condition to the parents, do we also remind parents that this baby would also still come with a full set of other human characteristics?' (Saxton 2000: 161). Here the disability rights critique centres on the 'failures of imagination' (Parens and Asch 2000b) of bioethicists, obstetricians and genetic counsellors to imagine disabled people might lead lives as valuable, rich and complex as their own, largely because of their lack of contact with disabled adults as equals and peers. Hence the recurring recommendation for more contact between members of the medical profession – including those in training – and disabled people, to increase the chances of the former having a more accurate and grounded understanding of the reality of the lives of the latter (Ralston 2000; Saxton 2000).

Prenatal testing and people with learning difficulties

For people with learning difficulties, their families and supporters, the issues surrounding prenatal testing are similar to those for other disabled people, but sharper in certain key areas.

First, the origins of most forms of learning disability have yet to be genetically determined and are only rarely attributable to inherited conditions (for example, Fragile X syndrome). Yet Down syndrome remains one of the two most frequent conditions tested for prenatally, with most tests followed by abortion, despite the fact that Down syndrome is not a life-threatening condition and many people with Down syndrome live full and happy lives. (It is, perhaps, significant that there is wide variation between different US states with regard to what constitutes 'serious' impairments, for which abortion should be available on Medicaid. In Iowa, for example, abortion is available for anenecephaly or severe, open spina bifida, but not Down syndrome 'which officials have decided is not sufficiently serious: Wertz 2000: 285).

Second, people with learning difficulties have tended to be marginal to the general disability movement, both within the United States and the United Kingdom, and, therefore, even less included in the debates in this area. They are disadvantaged here by their generally low level of literacy (and therefore acutely limited access to written materials on the subject) and less developed cognitive and verbal skills (which makes it hard for them to fill in for themselves the 'public silences' in this area – in particular, the non-explicit assumption that positive tests for impairment will be followed by abortion). In addition, there is the, perhaps understandable, assumption on the part of others that issues around genetics and prenatal testing are too complicated (not to mention too sensitive) both to explain and to understand (and indeed to handle, given the messages conveyed about society's lack of acceptance of people with Down syndrome, for example). So, for people with learning difficulties, the issue is much less 'The right to choose?' than the even more fundamental and basic 'Right to know'. This is, therefore, an area where much careful work still waits to be done.

One small, but ground-breaking, initiative undertaken in the United Kingdom took the form of a pair of linked workshops for eight people with learning difficulties, devised and run by two women in Bristol (Howarth and Rodgers 2001; Rodgers and Howarth 2001). A national information exchange on the subject of prenatal testing and people with learning difficulties was in the process of being organized, amid some concern on the part of the organizers, lest people with learning difficulties be excluded from both the event and related debates. Searching discussions confirmed the view that it would be inappropriate to invite people with learning difficulties to such an event without first giving them the opportunity to become clearly aware of the true, and multiple, issues involved. Two carefully constructed, accessible and participative, linked, day workshops resulted, with each participant given appropriate support, via the two organizers, an individual supporter already known to them (perhaps through where they lived), fellow attendees and the possibility of access to further, specialized, support (like counselling) if required.

The first workshop focused on *Difference and choice*, building up from discussions about 'Difference' (for example, having a learning difficulty) to consideration of how differences came about – culture, education, money, discrimination and . . . genes. This led on to a review of how babies were made, with flipchart illustrations, reinforced by further information for participants who were still unsure about some details. There was talk of what might be 'on people's genes' and things that might 'run in people's families', and whether learning difficulties was 'on a gene' or not. (Participants discovered that sometimes it was; sometimes it wasn't; and that sometimes you could find out in advance whether your baby was going to have a learning difficulty before she or he was born.)

The second workshop focused on *Choices*, beginning with where people lived, went on holiday, what they ate and so on. This built up to a discussion about 'Choices in pregnancy', that is, whether a woman might decide not to go through with having a baby, but to have an abortion instead. For some participants this was a completely new idea and needed to be gone over in some detail, with discussion in small groups of why people might make a decision of this kind and the sorts of pressures that might affect their decision. Not surprisingly, this was a difficult exercise for some people – not least, trying to understand why people might not want a baby with, for example, Down syndrome. There was a lot of debate about what it meant to be 'severely handicapped' (as the United Kingdom law puts it) and whether that made it all right to have an abortion, when you might not be able to in other circumstances. Then the workshop participants moved on to an exercise aimed at finding out what they thought about prenatal testing and abortion. Opinions were quite varied; for example: 'Tests are good because they give people information' and 'Disabled babies are OK'. Some indicated a clear grasp of the social context of disability: 'The foetus should be aborted if a test shows it has a learning difficulty because I don't think it should be born into a cruel world'; 'People with learning difficulties should be treated fairly and not discriminated against. Scientists should find the gene that makes people pick on those who are different. Then our lives would be better.'

The participants were asked what they thought would be useful for prospective parents who had been told that their foetus had an impairment and were trying to decide whether or not to have an abortion. They were clear that information about what people with learning difficulties *can* do would be helpful. And they felt strongly that people with learning difficulties should be involved in future debates about the use of genetic information to inform choices in pregnancy.

After the workshops the participants decided that they felt so strongly about what they had learnt that they wanted to present to the national conference to be held shortly afterwards. Their presentation proved to be the highlight of a day featuring contributions by leading commentators in the field of genetics, bioethics, research and disability and demonstrated persuasively that people with learning difficulties were quite capable of understanding and appreciating the complex issues involved in prenatal diagnosis in pregnancy and its social context, even if (like many of us) the specific clinical and scientific details of genetics and genetic technology were beyond them.

After the conference, the papers presented were written up for publication (Ward 2001). But another dilemma remained. The papers, though written relatively clearly, were certainly not accessible to most people with learning difficulties, who would not generally be able to read with any ease. There was a real risk that the book, while raising the profile of this hitherto neglected area, might still serve unwittingly to continue the exclusion of people with learning difficulties from the surrounding debate. Was it ethical to produce accessible information which might cause distress to people with learning difficulties (for example, learning that it was routine, even expected, in our society to opt for an abortion if the foetus had Down syndrome) or was it a greater injustice, and infringement of human rights, to deprive people with learning difficulties of access to information which affected them directly, but which they had hitherto been routinely denied? Eventually, the decision was taken to go ahead with the production of an easily understood, illustrated leaflet, based on the original workshops undertaken, refined after piloting with small groups of people with learning difficulties locally. The booklet was made available free, on request, to people with learning difficulties from the book publisher – with a prominent 'health warning' attached, to the effect that it was best read in conjunction with the support of a professional or someone else who would be at hand to talk through what might be painful discoveries (Howarth et al. 2001).

Conclusion

There are no simple conclusions to this chapter. The trend towards more and more prenatal testing (followed by abortion) is clear (Ossorio 2000). In the climate of litigation prevailing in the United States, for example, with the possibility of suits for 'wrongful life', 'wrongful birth' and 'infliction of emotional distress' by those affected by the birth of a disabled child, prenatal testing is set to become more, not less, widespread and routine. As Ossorio points out:

> The more tests physicians order to prevent liability, the more likely it is that they will create a legal duty to offer these tests, regardless of whether testing is otherwise well advised . . . If only a fraction of parents sue when their child is born with a disability but few or none sue when too many tests are done, the legal system will provide incentives for physicians to offer every feasible genetic test.
>
> (Ossorio 2000: 312)

The domination of the discourse by scientists, the medical profession and those with a commercial interest in the Human Genome Project and associated research continues. Though the public presentation of advances in genetic technology continues to focus on 'cures' and 'therapy' those accomplishments remain in the distant future. In the meantime, the social barriers facing people with learning difficulties (along with other disabled people) are exacerbated by their limited access to the kind of supports and services they need (at a cost of a fraction of the resources invested in genetic technology research) which are neither routinely, nor readily, available.

The assumption that society is 'better off without its disabled citizens' or at least those citizens born with an impairment (since only 1% of births are affected by congenital impairment, though 12% of the population is disabled: Shakespeare 2001) continues to be enshrined in the assumptions underpinning prenatal testing and abortion legislation in the United Kingdom. Those involved in genetic research fiercely reject any suggestion of 'eugenic' overtones to their work – yet it is hard to see how the desire for 'normality' and the 'perfect child', and the concomitant abhorrence of the different or the disabled, does not come from the same family of arguments as those only too publicly displayed in the twentieth century, most notably within Nazism but elsewhere too. While the rhetoric may be about the termination of pregnancies affected by 'severe handicap', the statistics show the dramatic fall in the birth rates of babies with much lesser impairments, for example cleft palates and talipes (club foot) (Alderson 2001). (See also, for instance, *BBC News Online*, 16 April 2004, on a legal challenge following the late abortion of a foetus with a cleft lip and palate, questioning how a cleft palate can be classed as a 'severe handicap' under abortion legislation.)

This chapter has concentrated on the implications of developments in prenatal testing for disabled people themselves, and people with learning difficulties in particular. Some of the problems experienced by some prospective parents as a result of the apparent increase in choice presented by more widespread prenatal testing have been referred to earlier, but many of the issues confronting (prospective) parents have not been rehearsed in detail. It is clear that the routinization of prenatal testing and genetic counselling is accepted and, indeed highly valued by some families, particularly those carrying a risk of an inherited disorder, like Fragile X syndrome (Carmichael 2003); that the provision of good counselling is a high priority for many working in this area (see Clarke 1994; Russell 2001) but that the availability of screening may itself generate some risk of adverse impact both on parents who subsequently give birth to a disabled child (after a false negative test result) and on attitudes to disability and disabled people generally (Hall et al 2000; Alderson 2001).

For the disability community (and its supporters) prenatal diagnosis, followed by abortion, is a social, moral and political issue, not simply a health or medical one, as traditionally perceived. 'Health professions have historically been the last, not the first, to adjust to the evolving interpretation of the meanings of disability in our society' (Ferguson et al. 2000: 87). Defining this as a 'human rights' issue, rather than a 'public health' one, makes it less easy to continue to hide the value judgements implicit here – the lack of worth ascribed to the lives of disabled people and the absence of a societal commitment to embracing diversity and difference – behind the spurious veneer of 'value-free' medical technology and scientific advancement. The risk, of course, is that widespread prenatal testing, often for impairments which are not life threatening and which are not incompatible with a good quality of life, 'engenders or reinforces public perceptions that the disabled should not exist, making intolerance and discrimination towards them more likely' (Robertson 1996). And it is hard to see how that message can sit easily with the official public commitment embodied in the United Kingdom's original Disability Discrimination Act 1995 (and the subsequent legislation to widen its scope), that discrimination against disabled people is not admissible and that disabled people are as equally valued as any other citizens.

References

Alderson, P. (2001) 'Unanswered questions', in L. Ward (ed.) *Considered Choices?* Kidderminster: British Institute of Learning Disabilities.

All Party Parliamentary Disablement Group (1999) 'Minutes of meeting of 19 October 1999 on genetics and disability', London: All Party Parliamentary Disablement Group (unpublished).

Bailey, R. (1996) 'Prenatal testing and the prevention of impairment: a woman's right to choose?', in J. Morris (ed.) *Encounters with Strangers: Feminism and Disability*. London: The Women's Press.

BBC News (2004) *Police Inquiry into Late Abortion*, http://news.bbc.co.uk/1/hi/england/hereford/worcs/3632169.stm (accessed 22 October 2004).

Biesecker, B.B. and Hamby, L. (2000) 'What difference the disability community arguments should make for the delivery of prenatal genetic information', in E. Parens and A. Asch (eds) *Prenatal Testing and Disability Rights*. Washington, DC: Georgetown University Press.

Carmichael, B. (2003) 'The Human Genome Project – threat or promise', *Journal of Intellectual Disability Research*, 47(7): 505–508.

Clarke, A. (1993) 'Is non-directive genetic counselling possible?', *Lancet*, 19 October: 998–1002.

Clarke, A. (ed.) (1994) *Genetic Counselling: Practice and Principles*. London: Routledge.

Disability Now (2000) 'Much ado about genetics', *Disability Now*, May: 1.

Disability Tribune (2000) Special issue on disability and bioethics, *Disability Tribune*, February. London: Disability Awareness in Action.

Disabled Peoples' International (DPI) – European Region (1998) *Bioethics and Disabled People: Proceedings of a Seminar*. London: DPI.

Dodds, R. (1997) *The Stress of Tests in Pregnancy: Summary of a National Childbirth Trust Antenatal Screening Survey*. London: National Childbirth Trust.

Ferguson, P., Gartner, A. and Lipsky, D. (2001) 'The experience of disability in families: a synthesis of research and parent narratives', in E. Parens and A. Asch (eds) *Prenatal Testing and Disability Rights*. Washington, DC: Georgetown University Press.

Finger, A. (1991) *Past Due: A Story of Disability, Pregnancy and Birth*. London: The Women's Press.

Fletcher, A. (1997) 'It's not the baby's responsibility to be perfect . . .', *Amazons*, newsletter of British Council of Disabled People (BCODP) Women's Group, June: 1, 4, 5.

Fletcher, A. (1999) *Genes are Us? Attitudes to Genetics and Disability: A RADAR Survey*. London: Royal Association for Disability and Rehabilitation (RADAR).

Fletcher, A. (2000) 'All Party Parliamentary Disablement Group Briefing on efforts to tackle genetic discrimination in the United States', London: All Party Parliamentary Disablement Group (unpublished).

Fletcher, A. (2001) 'Three generations of imbeciles are enough: eugenics, the new genetics and people with learning difficulties', in L. Ward (ed.) *Considered Choices?* Kidderminster: British Institute of Learning Disabilities.

Hall, S., Bobrow, M. and Marteau, T. (2000) 'Psychological consequences for parents of false negative results on prenatal screening for Down's Syndrome: retrospective interview study', *British Medical Journal*, 320: 407–412.

Herbert, S. (1997) '15,000 forcibly sterilised in France', *Daily Telegraph*, 11 September.

Howarth, J. and Rodgers, J. with others (2001) 'Difference and choice: a workshop for people with learning difficulties', in L. Ward (ed.), *Considered Choices?* Kidderminster: British Institute of Learning Disabilities.

Howarth, J., Rodgers, J. and Ward, L. (2001) *Difference and Choice*. Kidderminster: British Institute of Learning Disabilities, http://194.143.187.101/index.htm (accessed 22 October 2004).

Institute of Medicine (Committee on Assessing Genetic Risks, Division of Health Sciences Policy) (1994) *Assessing Genetic Risks: Implications for Health and Social Policy*. Washington, DC: National Academy Press.

Jennings, B. (2000) 'Technology and the genetic imaginary: prenatal testing and the construction of disability', in E. Parens and A. Asch (eds) *Prenatal Testing and Disability Rights*. Washington, DC: Georgetown University Press.

Kaplan, D. (1994) 'Prenatal screening and diagnosis: the impact on persons with disabilities', in K. Rothenberg and E. Thomson (eds) *Women and Prenatal Testing*. Columbus, OH: Ohio State University Press.

Morris, J. (1991) *Pride against Prejudice: Transforming Attitudes to Disability*. London: The Women's Press.

Morris, J. (1996) 'Introduction', in J. Morris (ed.) *Encounters with Strangers: Feminism and Disability*. London: The Women's Press.

Ossorio, P. (2000) 'Prenatal genetic testing and the courts', in E. Parens and A. Asch (eds) *Prenatal Testing and Disability Rights*. Washington, DC: Georgetown University Press.

Parens, E. and Asch, A. (eds) (2000a) *Prenatal Testing and Disability Rights*. Washington, DC: Georgetown University Press.

Parens, E. and Asch, A. (2000b) 'The disability rights critique of prenatal genetic testing: reflections and recommendations', in E. Parens and A. Asch (eds) *Prenatal Testing and Disability Rights*. Washington, DC: Georgetown University Press.

Press, N. (2000) 'Assessing the expressive character of prenatal testing: the choices made or the choices made available?', in E. Parens and A. Asch (eds) *Prenatal Testing and Disability Rights*. Washington, DC: Georgetown University Press.

Ralston, S. (2000) 'Reflections from the trenches: one doctor's encounter with disability rights arguments', in E. Parens and A. Asch (eds) *Prenatal Testing and Disability Rights*. Washington, DC: Georgetown University Press.

Rioux, M. (2001) 'The many interests in genetic knowledge: an international perspective on prenatal screening and the use of genetic information in relation to people with learning difficulties', in L. Ward (ed.) *Considered Choices?* Kidderminster: British Institute of Learning Disabilities.

Robertson, J.A. (1996) 'Genetic selection of offspring characteristics', *Boston University Law Review*, 76(3): 421–482.

Rodgers, J. and Howarth, J. (2001) 'Difference and choice: helping people with learning difficulties to consider ethical issues around genetics', in L. Ward (ed.) *Considered Choices?* Kidderminster: British Institute of Learning Disabilities.

Rothenberg, K. and Thomson, E. (eds) (1994) *Women and Prenatal Testing: Facing the Challenges of Genetic Technology*. Columbus, OH: Ohio State University Press.

Rothman, B.K. (1984) 'The meanings of choice in reproductive technology', in R. Arditti, R. Duelli Klein and S. Minden (eds) *Test Tube Women: What Future for Motherhood?* London: Pandora.

Russell, O. (2001) 'Supporting families to make informed choices: how can we safeguard genetic diversity while respecting parents' "right to choose"?', in L. Ward (ed.) *Considered Choices?* Kidderminster: British Institute of Learning Disabilities.

Saxton, M. (2000) 'Why members of the disability community oppose prenatal diagnosis and selective abortion', in E. Parens and A. Asch (eds) *Prenatal Testing and Disability Rights*. Washington, DC: Georgetown University Press.

Shakespeare, T. (1998) 'Disability and genetics', in Disabled Peoples' International – European Region, *Bioethics and Disabled People*. London: DPI.

Shakespeare, T. (2000) 'Genetics research and disabilities: what are the issues?' (unpublished).

Shakespeare, T. (2001) 'Foreword', in L. Ward (ed.) *Considered Choices?* Kidderminster: British Institute of Learning Disabilities.

Sutherland, A. (1981) *Disabled We Stand*. London: Souvenir Press.

Ward, L. (ed.) (2001) *Considered Choices? The New Genetics, Prenatal Testing and People with Learning Disabilities*. Kidderminster: British Institute of Learning Disabilities.

Wertz, D. (2000) 'Drawing lines: notes for policy-makers', in E. Parens and A. Asch (eds) *Prenatal Testing and Disability Rights*. Washington, DC: Georgetown University Press.

Williams, C. (1997) *Terminus Brain: The Environmental Threats to Human Intelligence*. London: Cassell.

Chapter 8

'New' genetics meets the old underclass

Findings from a study of genetic outreach services in rural Kentucky

Susan E. Kelly

Introduction

One of the most serious, but least examined, issues arising at the intersection of the 'new' genetics and public health is the relationship between social class and genetic burden. In the United States, concerns in ethics, policy and public discourses about genetic medicine and class structure have frequently been expressed in the notion of a potential 'genetic underclass' (Nelkin and Tancredi 1989; Lee 1993; Mehlman and Botkin 1998). In general outline, the genetic underclass is conceptualized as an economically segregated, biologically inferior, socially and politically marginalized status emerging from inequities of access to genetic health benefits or genetic enhancements. Genetic underclass formation is predicted by some to occur through such mechanisms as genetic discrimination in employment and insurance, and following from the use of genetic knowledge and technologies within existing mechanisms of class division and social oppression. Drawn loosely from debates about the underclass in sociological theories of stratification, the genetic underclass notion intermingles threats of stigma, deviance and economic displacement. 'Culture of poverty' explanations of underclass persistence emphasize that the stigma of undeservingness and marginality is passed on to future generations, recalling eugenic social ideologies in which the stigma of 'bad' genes was seen similarly to have been passed on.

The goal of this chapter is to offer a new perspective on the genetic underclass metaphor. I draw from research conducted on a public health genetic outreach programme serving a geographically disadvantaged population in the United States. I will first briefly consider the notion of the genetic underclass as it has appeared in medical ethics and policy literatures, and argue that the mechanisms of access and discrimination which are associated with the genetic underclass concept are not likely to be those through which the new genetics will most forcefully intersect with social disadvantage. Little direct evidence currently exists to substantiate a genetically unemployable or uninsurable underclass; rather, this notion is based on the assumption that genetic knowledge and services are different in significant ways from other medical services, and reflects little of the complex structural creation and persistence of class. However, theoretical dimensions associated with the underclass as it appears in social stratification literature do suggest ways of examining dynamics of genetic conditions and social disadvantage. In the second section of the chapter, drawing from analyses of research cases, I identify issues and processes that will be of importance to understanding relationships between social disadvantage and genetics.

Theories of a genetic underclass

The term 'underclass' appears to have been introduced into the literature by Myrdal (1944) to describe an emergent substratum of the American population that was structurally excluded from larger economic processes of society, its members characterized as the permanently unemployed, the unemployable and the underemployed. Sociological theories of the emergence and persistence of an underclass argue the relative contributions of cultural values attributed to disadvantaged groups, economic and political structures, and individual genetic endowment. Cultural explanations generally argue that a distinctive, culturally determined way of life largely explains the occurrence and persistence of poverty. Values such as a limited time horizon, low aspirations and impulsive need for gratification comprise a world-view into which succeeding generations are socialized; this culture of poverty limits individuals' abilities to participate in mainstream institutions (Albrecht et al. 2000), and leads to breakdown in family structure (e.g. marital dissolution, illegitimacy). The 'defective' set of values and norms helps people cope with the pervasive hopelessness and despair of poverty but locks the underclass into a permanent, maladaptive culture.

Structural explanations seek the causes of poverty in the social or economic system. Discrimination and segregation resulting from racism and sexism, and economic restructuring since the Second World War are argued to have resulted in the economic and social marginalization of entire groups of people. Wilson (1987) linked the emergence of an urban underclass to historical discrimination, mass migration of African Americans to northern cities in the first half of the twentieth century, and subsequent industrial and geographic restructuring of urban economies since the 1960s. A competing conservative sociological underclass discourse (notably Murray 1994, 1999) argues that the underclass comprises those who are poor by choice, demotivated by social welfare programmes, influenced by bad role models, and characterized by deviant behaviour (e.g. illegitimate births) and lack of personal responsibility.

Underclass or social exclusion discourses, since the 1980s, have had considerable currency in political disputes about income distribution, racial/ethnic segregation, education policies and health (Andersen 1999).

The conservative discourse in these debates has increasingly assumed an intrinsic, biogenic character (Rothenberg and Heinz 1998). (See, for example, Lewontin et al. 1984, for a discussion of the confluent resurgence of conservative social policy discourse and the new genetics.) Conceptual implications of underclass dimensions such as social segregation, polarization and exclusion (Mohan 2000) to describe effects of unequal access to or application of genetic knowledge and technologies are widely appealing. Exclusion, for example, has been applied broadly to refer to those unable to participate in society principally for non-economic, health-based reasons such as mental illness, physical incapacity, or old age, but has also been applied narrowly to refer principally to non-participation in paid employment (the major source of private health insurance coverage in the United States). However, genetic underclass arguments appearing in the US literature on social implications of the new genetics as yet merely draw from evocative terminology associated with the underclass concept, without engaging causal debates within stratification research, particularly those concerning intrinsic or extrinsic factors or structural and cultural dynamics.

Current usage of the genetic underclass concept may be traced to Nelkin and Tancredi's use of the term 'biologic underclass' in the book *Dangerous Diagnostics: The Social Power of Biological Information* (1989). Explanations for the emergence of a genetic underclass in the recent US literature emphasize two mechanisms: genetic discrimination (primarily through workplace and health insurance) and unequal access to and use of genetic medicine and enhancement technologies. The first category of explanation, genetic discrimination, locates the emergence of a genetic underclass at the juncture of the increasing development of genetic technologies and information, and rational business practices. Particularly in the United States there has been significant concern that risk-rating practices within the insurance industry will inevitably exploit the predictive and discriminatory potential of genetic information to exclude and disenfranchise individuals on the basis of information to be gained through genetic testing (e.g. Gostin 1991; Hudson et al. 1997). Employers have strong incentives to require employees to reveal, through medical records or testing, any genetic traits that may make them more vulnerable to work hazards or more costly to insure (Draper 1992). The result, it is claimed, may be a 'class' of biological undesirables excluded from occupations and health services on the basis of genetic make-up (Lee 1993; O'Hara 1993).

Laws in many US states prohibit insurers from denying coverage on the basis that a genetic risk represents a pre-existing condition. Although no current federal legislation has been passed directly relating to genetic discrimination in individual insurance or in the workplace, the Health Insurance Portability and Accountability Act of 1996 forbids group health insurers from taking such actions (Reilly 2001). At least thirty-two states have passed laws prohibiting genetic discrimination in employment (NCSL 2004). However, in a review of legislation and insurance underwriting activity (Reilly 2001: 268), little evidence was found that genetic information to date has been used to deny health insurance or employment. Hall and Rich (2000) found virtually no well-documented cases of health insurers either asking for or using presymptomatic genetic test results in their underwriting decisions, before or after non-discrimination laws had been enacted, and in states with or without such laws. They concluded that a person with a serious genetic condition who is presymptomatic faces little or no difficulty in obtaining private health insurance. The researchers concluded that existence of the laws may influence how industry perceives the legitimacy of using genetic information and thus provide a deterrent to future discriminatory practices. In the area of employment discrimination, the Equal Employment Opportunities Commission (EEOC) issued a guideline interpreting the Americans with Disabilities Act (ADA) of 1990 as forbidding the use of genetic information in hiring or promotion (Reilly 2001). However, this protection has not undergone substantial judicial scrutiny and only one lawsuit (a successful suit against the Burlington Northern and Santa Fe Railway) has been filed to date by the EEOC on behalf of workers (Lewin 2001).

Possible barriers that currently may be preventing legitimate cases of genetic discrimination from coming forward under the ADA remain to be investigated, but may include that negative pressures exist within industry sufficient to prevent persons experiencing genetic discrimination from seeking available forms of protection, and/or that discrimination that is based on genetic information and is distinct from other forms of employment discrimination is not occurring to a significant degree. However, examination of current patterns of use of genetic information in industry does not support the emergence of a significant strata or class of the genetically undesirable and unemployable.

The second category of explanation of a genetic underclass is invoked in discussions of social implications of genetic medicine and genetic enhancement. In these contexts, existing class inequalities, particularly those of income, education and quality of medical care that are related to inequalities in access to medical treatments are predicted to lead to inequalities in biology (Mehlman and Botkin 1998). According to this argument, these disparities will lead to a 'widening gulf between the genetically privileged and the genetic underclass' (Mehlman and Botkin 1998: 99). Wealthy parents will select and purchase 'biological advantages' for/in their offspring including freedom from genetic disease, intelligence and beauty, while those on the other side of the deepening class divide will continue to suffer from genetic illness and with less effective, conventional medical treatments and methods of self-improvement. However, fears that unequal access to genetic technologies will produce substantial biological differences among classes, beyond currently existing disparities in health status, may exaggerate the potential of single-gene disease treatment or enhancement technologies

(Holtzman and Marteau 2000). Such fears further reflect an assumption that genuine advances in health care following from genetic research, rather than affecting overall changes in clinical practice, will impact health care delivery in significantly segmented ways. One area in which health effects may be segmented is the widespread use of reproductive genetic technologies including assisted reproduction and prenatal screening and testing for genetic conditions or traits (e.g., Kupperman et al. 1996; Khoshnood et al. 2000). However, little evidence exists that these practices alone are creating significant health disparities above differences in access to and quality of prenatal care, environmental exposures, and other factors related to socio-economic status. In addition, while coverage of novel treatments in their early stages is frequently denied by private and public insurers, access may be vigorously and successfully pursued through legal and other avenues of redress (Kelly and Koenig 1998). Consumer lobbying and other advocacy efforts for screening and/or treatment of genetic diseases such as Tay-Sachs disease, galactosaemia and sickle-cell anaemia have been successful (Reilly 1977; Rapp 1999; Duster 2003).

Public health genetics: rural outreach programmes

Rural outreach programmes for genetic services in the United States were developed to address inequalities of access to genetic counselling, testing, and expertise that exist on the basis of material, social, and geographic disadvantage. Initiated with federal funding in 1978, outreach programmes currently exist in all fifty states, District of Columbia, Puerto Rico and the Virgin Islands. The extent to which such programmes solve problems of access or quality of genetic services provided to socially and medically disadvantaged populations has received little examination (but see Marfatia et al. 1990; Coffman et al. 1993; Trottier and Crandall 1996; Dobie et al. 1998; Mitchell and Petroski 1998). In Kentucky, genetic outreach services are provided by two university medical centre based teams who hold on-site clinics in county public health facilities across the state. Services provided include reproductive genetic counselling, genetic diagnosis and follow-up for primarily paediatric patients with genetic or congenital conditions. Geneticists refer patients for medical services locally as well as to specialists at the state's two university-based medical centres. In fiscal year 2000, 1335 clients received genetic outreach services (Davis 2001).

The study

The purpose of this study was to provide information about state efforts to improve access to genetic services through examination of the genetic outreach programme in Kentucky, a substantially rural state with significant geographic disparities in access to medical care and health professionals. The broader question to which this study was addressed is the nature of interactions between social disadvantage and genetics. How does a genetic diagnosis and/or genetic condition interact with life circumstances, in particular the systems and institutions through which genetics is made socially meaningful? Data were collected as part of a three-year, qualitative study of access, use and experiences of genetic services among parents living in primarily rural counties outside the two major metropolitan areas of the state.

Methods

The methodology used in the study was qualitative, with data being collected primarily through in-depth, semi-structured interviews. Interview subjects were guided through a set of question areas that were standardized but employed with flexibility to identify and explore issues of importance to subjects' experiences and to incorporate insights thus gained into the research process. Interviews were conducted with eighty parents (all but three being mothers) of children who are clients of a rural genetic outreach clinic. Interviews explored experiences related to prenatal care and childbirth, diagnosis and use of health care services. Employment, family support, transportation and insurance information were also collected. Respondents reflected the racial/ethnic demographics of rural portions of the state; all but three were White. The median age was 30–39 and the median annual household income was $20,000 to $50,000. The majority was married, either not employed outside the home or employed part-time, and held either a high-school or equivalency degree and some technical training. Four brief case studies provide insight into the patterns of dynamics identified in the data, through which social disadvantage and the burden of genetic disease might constitute mutually reinforcing processes in the make up of a 'genetic underclass'. In contrast to most previous studies of genetic services, the focus of the present study is not on a particular genetic condition or form of testing, but rather on a wide range of common and rare genetic conditions and the broader bundle of genetic services provided in a public health setting.

Cumulative disadvantage

The lives of individuals and families in all four cases were affected by interrelationships of genetics, social position, geo-spatial location and health and social service structures that tended to accumulate in constant downward pressure on life circumstances.[1] No respondent reported any form of genetic discrimination or denial of insurance, employment or services on the basis of genetic information or disease. Rather, the data demonstrate forms of social disadvantage following from specific genetic manifestations and discrimination related to disability and poverty more generally; these formed significant barriers and negative pressures in the lives of the majority of families. For many in the study, the birth of a child with a genetic condition has been followed by a constant struggle against forces that impact on educational and employment opportunities, household finances and mobility, family structure and behaviour – all dimensions associated with the underclass concept.

Ann

Ann, the mother of a son affected with a rare, severely disabling genetic condition and two non-affected children, exemplifies the interaction of social and structural factors that may result in cumulative disadvantage. While in some ways less socially disadvantaged than many of the people in the study, Ann is engaged in constant struggle against forces of marginalization affecting herself and her family. She maintains a financially precarious existence requiring constant efforts to piece together – and balance – earned income, state assistance, private and public insurance, and medical and social services. The patchwork has holes: although her affected son and one of his siblings are covered by a private insurance policy held by Ann's first husband, neither she nor her third child from a second marriage are covered by any private or public form of insurance. Nonetheless, she finds the financial burden associated with her affected child's care tremendous, due to high out-of-pocket costs and uncovered expenses. Ann's ability to work is constrained by the severity of her son's impairment and her status as a single mother (a status she attributes to the emotional and financial strains of caring for her son). In the following quotations she discusses the cumulative pressure of her single status, the requirements of her child's medical needs, and the misfit of available services to her life circumstances and needs:

> County Family Services has respite care and it amounts to, I'm going to guess, between 500 and 800 dollars a month for Sam. And the way that it works is you find the respite provider. So it could be my mother or a neighbour and then you pay them out of your own pocket. And then you send in a reimbursement form and they will pay you back. And the problem I have with that . . . I couldn't ask a neighbour to babysit. Well, I don't have a neighbour, for one thing. I'm in a very rural community, we're way out in the country. It's not like living in town where your neighbours get to know you and see you with Sam . . . They know that he's here, but they don't know anything about him and wouldn't be comfortable with keeping him. But it would be difficult to get them to babysit and then tell them I'll pay them later because . . . I don't have 50 or 60 dollars at the drop of a hat just to give to someone and wait four weeks for that to come back to me.

> And, financially is where they [her other children] really feel it because I don't work much outside the home, and when I do I don't make a whole lot of money. It's important for me to go to work after Sam gets on the school bus and then I need to be here when he gets home . . . But what that does is limit me from going downtown and leaving at 7, getting off at 5, there is no way that I could do that because there is no one here to put Sam on and off the bus . . . My 13 year old could probably manage it but the district or the county does not allow the bus drivers to pick them up or release them to anyone but an adult.

In Ann's circumstances, her child's condition demands complex, skilled caregiving that she feels uncomfortable turning over to others; nor are others comfortable providing respite care. Although the school district provides transportation to school, Ann finds herself limited in her employment options by the need to be at home when her affected child is put on the bus in the morning and returns home in the afternoon. She is caught in gaps between the distinctive needs of her affected child, and the limits of public services available to support her.

Cumulative disadvantage is manifest socially as well. Ann discusses the effects of their life conditions on her other two children.

> My other two children are going to be 14 and 15 and they're going to be going off somewhere to college or maybe somewhere, and there is nothing for them you know. The new bikes aren't here, the new shoes, the Reeboks, the Nikes. The times that people have told them they're poor I can't even tell you . . . the little boy next door . . . he found out about that, he saw the shoes one day, and that was it, you all are poor, you're poor white trash. You're poor white trash.

Alice

The inadequacies of private insurance in the face of constant and significant medical needs are common among families in the study and are directly tied to ability to earn income. Alice and her partner filed for bankruptcy shortly after their first child Robert was born with a rare genetic condition resulting in skeletal malformation, even though the insurance policy provided through her partner's employment had a maximum of $250,000 per year for dependants. The insurance

> paid its limit, Lord yes . . . well man, it hit us by the time he was 4 months old. We'd done went past $250,000. So we had no insurance . . . Robert was a year old when we filed bankruptcy . . . You know, you do what you've got to do.

Alice's current employment as an instructional assistant through the county Board of Education does not provide private health insurance for herself or her other two children. Although the genetic outreach personnel (and two university medical centres) have not yet been able to provide a definitive diagnosis for Robert 's condition, they were eventually able to assist Alice in obtaining Medicaid coverage for Robert by the time he was 2 years old. The medical card 'has been a lifesaver', covering most of the expenses associated with Robert's condition; however, for the intervening period Alice and her family received financial and other material support from churches and neighbours in her rural community. Like a number of families in the study, Alice and her partner are not formally living together or married because he no longer has private health insurance through his employer (he is employed by a small company not covered by regulations requiring that private health insurance plans be offered; the company dropped him from their insurance after the expenses of Robert 's initial 4 months of life) and their combined incomes would disqualify Robert for state medical assistance. In Kentucky, 47.5 per cent of low-income families (defined as income below 200 per cent of the 2003 Federal Poverty Guidelines or $37,320 for a family of four) are uninsured (Families USA 2004). Also like other families in the study, the severity and development of their child's genetic condition impose medical requirements that simply could not be met without state-provided insurance coverage. Income eligibility is an imperative, and is maintained by strategies with implications for family stability and socioeconomic status including not taking advancement at work, working part-time or becoming unemployed, and fictitious or 'paper' marital dissolution. The inability to marry in spite of raising a family of three children goes deeply against Alice's religious beliefs and community norms, induces shame, and contributes substantially to the stresses under which she lives.

Hannah

Hannah, single mother of a teenage daughter, Nicole, affected with neurological and physical impairments, forgoes seeking medical care for complication of her own illness problems resulting from Type 1 diabetes. The co-payment of $35 per visit required under her private health insurance plan is unmanageable on a salary of $8.50 per hour for part-time work in the school district. Her health has severely deteriorated over the past several years, complicated by untreated asthma, degrading her ability to work. In addition, after the birth of her child, who required multiple surgeries and extensive medical care, she was unable to obtain Supplemental Security Income (SSI) disability payments for two years.

> They just kept denying her. Even though they knew about all of the medical problems she has . . . they just kept denying her. Said she didn't qualify and . . .

> because of my gross income. I mean in 1987 I wasn't making even four dollars an hour you know. And they just said, they didn't have enough medical information.

In Hannah's case as well, intervention by the outreach programme geneticist was required to obtain state assistance. For most parents, difficulties in manoeuvring one's way through 'the system', locating available programmes, and 'understanding one's rights' were central themes.

Ann's experience is typical:

> Not just genetic counselling services but a full range of things, a full range . . . I think of the services that would not have been available to Sam had it been – had I not asked for them. You know, being in the physician's office and listening to what they have to say, as they're walking out the door if I had not said, wait a minute, what about this or what about that. Oh yes, we do have those services . . . They know about it but it wasn't given to me until I asked for it.

Lily

Lily, single mother of a child, Abby, with Angelman's syndrome, sat on the couch in her darkened living room during our interview and held her daughter. At 10 years old, she is still in diapers and cannot walk – Lily through some miracle is still able to carry her. She is exhausted, having come home at midnight from working the third shift at a local assembly plant. Her daughter had recently suffered a seizure that threw her from her highchair and into the kitchen cabinet, breaking her collarbone. Lily drove her to the emergency room in a community about 30 minutes from her rural home. She has recently returned to paid employment after a number of years on public assistance. A home health aide had been watching her while Lily worked. However, the local agency that provides home health aides in Lily's community does not have enough staff to continue to send someone out to watch Abby while Lily works; while chronic and disabling, her condition is not considered life threatening. With staff and funding cutbacks and difficulty attracting trained ancillary health care workers to the county, the agency performs 'triage'. Lily is trying to figure out how to take leave from her new job, temporarily, to care for her daughter although there is no evidence that her problem will be anything but permanent. Although she has a partner, they are not able to marry and do not live together, again in order to protect Abby's eligibility for assistance. Although her parents live nearby, they also work second shift in the factory and are unable to provide regular child care.

Abby's father left the family shortly after her birth and does not pay child support. Abby's medical care is covered by Medicaid; although Lily works, her income is low enough to qualify her to receive Medicaid. However, many expenses associated with Abby's condition were not covered for the five years it took until Lily was able to receive a referral for genetic evaluation and diagnosis. Limited medical knowledge and lack of diffusion of expertise about genetic conditions result in delayed and inaccurate diagnoses for many parents, causing delayed entry into state medical and rehabilitative assistance and further exacerbating the financial and emotional burden of ill-health and disability. Lily attributes this delay to unfamiliarity with Angelman's and other genetic conditions within the paediatric community, her status as a single Medicaid mother, and unwillingness of Abby's physicians to make a diagnosis. With the genetic diagnosis, Lily gained access to SSI and other state-provided services.

The cases presented here encompass problems faced by many parents of children with severe genetic conditions in the study. Many of these families have moved into or are trapped in low incomes in spite of constant struggle to keep their families in the mainstream, battling funding agencies, school districts, specialist medical services, medical equipment providers, home health agencies and respite providers. Many families not only have depleted their savings but also live with greatly reduced income to allow one parent to take on the full-time responsibility of caregiving and paperwork. Family stresses include emotional and financial anxieties over lifelong care, social reaction and stigma, need to travel to received specialty medical services and uncertainty of future prognosis (Yanzti et al. 2001). Manifestations of these challenges and the contribution of genetics to overall burden and cumulative disadvantage are generally underexamined in academic and public discussions of the social implications of the new genetics.

Conclusion

By focusing on the mechanisms of genetic discrimination and inequalities of access to genetic treatment and enhancement technologies, the use of the underclass metaphor loses much of its analytic potential. Sociologically, theories of the underclass point to cumulative dynamics of social disadvantage, geo-spatial and social forms of segregation and exclusion, and above all, marginality and structural barriers to participation in the mainstream. I argue that although suggestive, the contexts in which the genetic underclass is invoked are not likely to be those that capture significant dynamics between social disadvantage and genetic burden. Nor is evidence available from which to draw conclusions about the implications of sporadic genetic discrimination in these settings and the formation of new genetically based social groups of the persistently excluded, marginalized and poor.

Although limited in scope, this analysis points to interactive processes among genetics (the lived experience of a genetic condition and clinical availability of genetic services and expertise) and social and structural forces including policy and social services, rural and class economic disadvantage, and social exclusion. To the extent a genetic underclass exists or may come to exist, it may be constituted through cumulative stresses on the lives of families resulting from factors including poorly co-ordinated, underfunded, and punitive health and social service structures, stresses that may encourage family disruption, unemployment, and reliance on vulnerable state-provided health insurance. Significantly at a time when major changes in federal health programmes are being debated, families of children with genetic conditions that involve chronic, severe and/or uncommon health care and other physical and developmental needs are most poorly served by state assistance and private insurance structures that are designed to discourage 'inappropriate' or 'frivolous' use of services, because their needs for medical care are inflexible. Cutbacks in the political economy of governance often target services for genetic diseases, which have a very low priority when compared to more pressing maternal or child health needs (Rapp 1999). It is significant that access to genetic services through the genetic outreach programme plays a range of roles in the lives of client families, including providing diagnoses, reassurance and, importantly, assistance in identifying and accessing state health insurance and other service programmes.

These findings point to the need to identify ways in which the experience of genetic conditions may differ from other forms of illness or disability, particularly chronic illness, and the specific ways in which a genetic underclass may be distinguished from a 'health' underclass more generally. At the present time, urban/rural disparities in the availability of genetic expertise, and uneven familiarity with genetic conditions among medical professionals and service providers, present a specific set of problems for families experiencing a genetic condition or disease. These include delays in receiving a diagnosis, contributing to inappropriate or delayed treatment and delayed entry into state-provided service programmes (see Sloper and Turner 1992). Rare conditions often present families with a complex and uncertain prognosis with which available medical services can provide little guidance and assistance. The relative lack of assistance from the medical community for rare conditions places an additional burden of care on families. Obtaining specialist treatment for rare genetic conditions may involve travel out of state; the costs associated with such travel can be both devastating and prohibitive. Difficulty locating respite and childcare services competent and willing to take on a child with exceptional health, dietary or behavioural requirements (e.g. Prader-Willi syndrome) contributes further emotional and financial stress. These difficulties extend to struggles to receive services within the educational system. These data indicate that severe genetic conditions may impact family members in ways that may invoke guilt, fear and/or shame, complicating family relationships and the provision of family support.

From a policy perspective, sustained attention should be paid to the overall location of families with genetic disabilities in terms of the specifics of their geography, economics, employment and access to health services and insurance. Individuals and families living in rural and medically underserved areas are particularly vulnerable to lack of adequate private and public medical insurance, social isolation, limited employment opportunities, insufficient supply of service providers, and limited, uneven existence and politics of resource distribution at the local level. Genetic disability may present families with issues of unfamiliarity, uncertainty, interfamilial difficulty and stigma, which may undermine the sense of efficacy and agency required to sustain efforts to keep lives from constantly being pushed further to the margins. These constitute a particularly onerous burden that may contribute significantly to a 'genetic underclass', beyond issues of access to technology and genetic discrimination in employment and insurance.

Acknowledgements

This research was supported by the National Human Genome Research Institute, R01 HG01975-01. I wish to thank the physicians and genetic counsellors who provided access to the genetic outreach programmes, and the parents who so generously agreed to participate in the study.

Note

1 To protect privacy and maintain anonymity, cases are presented using pseudonyms and with some alteration of non-essential demographic detail.

References

Albrecht, D.E., Albrecht, C.M. and Albrecht, S.L. (2000) 'Poverty in nonmetropolitan areas: impacts of industrial, employment, and family structure variables', *Rural Sociology*, 65(1): 87–103.

Andersen, J. (1999) 'Post-industrial solidarity or meritocracy?', *Acta Sociologica*, 42: 375–385.

Coffman, M.A., Kinney, S.K., Shissler, J.N., Leuthard, J.L. and DePersio, S.R. (1993) 'Reproductive genetic services in rural Oklahoma', *Fetal Diagnosis and Therapy*, 8(Suppl. 1): 128–141.

Davis, S. (2001) 'Genetic services in Kentucky'. Presented at *Genetics in Kentucky: Preparing for the Future*. Sponsored by the Cabinet for Health Services, Department of Public Health, Frankfort, KY, 1 May.

Dobie, S.A., Gorber, L. and Rosenblatt, R.A. (1998) 'Family planning service provision in rural areas: a survey in Washington State', *Family Planning Perspectives*, 30(3): 139–142, 147.

Draper, E. (1992) 'Genetic secrets: social issues of medical screening in a genetic age', *Hastings Center Report*, 22(4, suppl): S15–S18.

Duster, T. (2003) *Backdoor to Eugenics*. New York: Routledge.

Families USA (2004) 'The uninsured: a closer look. Kentuckians without health insurance', http://www.familiesusa.org/site/DocServer/kentucky.pdf?docID=3712 (accessed 30 November 2004).

Gostin, L. (1991) 'Genetic discrimination: the use of genetically based diagnostic and prognostic tests by employers and insurers', *American Journal of Law and Medicine*, 17(1–2): 109–144.

Hall, M.A. and Rich, S.S. (2000) 'Laws restricting health insurers' use of genetic information: impact on genetic discrimination', *American Journal of Human Genetics*, 66(1): 293–308.

Holtzman, N.A. and Marteau, T.M. (2000) 'Will genetics revolutionize medicine?' *New England Journal of Medicine*, 343(2): 141–144.

Hudson, K.L., Rothenberg, K.H., Andrews, L.B., Khan, M.J.E. and Collins, F.S. (1995) 'Genetic discrimination and health insurance: an urgent need for reform', *Science*, 270: 391–393.

Kelly, S.E. and Koenig, B.A. (1998) 'Rescue technologies following high dose chemotherapy for breast cancer: how social context shapes the assessment of innovative, aggressive, and life-saving medical technologies', in P.J. Boyle (ed) *Getting Doctors to Listen: Ethics and Outcomes Data in Context*. Washington, DC: Georgetown University Press.

Khoshnood, B., Pryde, P., Wall, S., Singh, J. Mittendorf, R. and Lee, K.S. (2000) 'Ethnic differences in the impact of advanced maternal age on birth prevalence of Down Syndrome', *American Journal of Public Health*, 90(11): 1778–1781.

Kuppermann, M., Gates, E. and Washington, A.E. (1996) 'Racial/ethnic differences in prenatal diagnostic test use and outcomes: preferences, socioeconomics, or patient knowledge?' *Obstetrics & Gynecology*, 87(5, Part 1): 675–682.

Lee, C. (1993) 'Creating a genetic underclass: the potential for genetic discrimination by the health insurance industry', *Pace Law Review*, 13(1): 189–228.

Lewin, T. (2001) 'Commission sues railroad to end genetic testing in work injury cases', *The New York Times*: 10 February.

Lewontin, R.C., Rose, S. and Kamin, L.J. (1984) *Not in our Genes: Biology, Ideology, and Human Nature*. New York: Pantheon.

Lippman, A. (1991) 'Prenatal genetic testing and screening: constructing needs and reinforcing inequities', *American Journal of Law and Medicine*, 17(1–2): 15–50.

Marfatia, L., Punjales-Morejon, D. and Rapp, R. (1990) 'Counseling the underserved: when an old reproductive technology becomes a new reproductive technology', in B.A. Fine, E. Getting, K. Greendale, B. Leopold and N. Rals (eds) *Strategies in Genetic Counseling: Reproductive Genetics and New Technologies*. White Plains, NY: March of Dimes Birth Defects Foundation.

Mehlman, M.J. and Botkin, J.R. (1998) *Access to the Genome: The Challenge to Equality*. Washington, DC: Georgetown University Press.

Mitchell, J.A. and Petroski, G. (1998) 'Evaluation of a statewide program in genetic diseases', *American Journal of Medicine Genetics*, 78: 217–225.

Mohan, J. (2000) 'Geographies of welfare and social exclusion', *Progress in Human Geography*, 24(2): 291–300.

Murray, C. (1994) *Losing Ground: American Social Policy, 1950–1980*. New York: Basic Books.

Murray, C. (1999) 'And now for the bad news', *Society*, 37(1): 12–15.

Myrdal, G. (1944) *An American Dilemma: The Negro Problem and Modern Democracy*. New York: Harper and Brothers.

National Conference of State Legislatures (2004) State Genetic Employment Laws. Available at http://www.nscl.org/programs/health/genetics/ndiscrim.htm (accessed 21 October 2004).

Nelkin, D. and Tancredi, L. (1989) *Dangerous Diagnostics: The Social Power of Biological Information*. New York: Basic Books.

O'Hara, S. (1993) 'The use of genetic testing in the health insurance industry: the creation of a "biologic underclass"', *Southwestern University Law Review*, 22(4): 1211–1228.

Rapp, R. (1999) *Testing Women, Testing the Fetus: The Social Impact of Amniocentesis in America*. New York and London: Routledge.

Reilly, P.R. (1977) *Genetics, the Law and Social Policy*. Cambridge, MA: Harvard University Press.

Reilly, P.R. (2001) 'Legal issues in genomic medicine', *Nature Medicine*, 7(3): 268–271.

Rothenberg, J. and Heinz, A. (1998) 'Meddling with monkey metaphors – capitalism and the threat of impulsive desires', *Social Justice*, 25(2): 44–64.

Sloper, P. and Turner, S. (1992) 'Service needs of families of children with severe physical disabilities', *Child: Care, Health and Development*, 18: 259–282.

Trottier, R.W. and Crandall, L.A. (1996) 'Public sector genetic services in Florida and Georgia: current status and potential issues raised by the Human Genome Project', Final Report to US Department of Energy DE-FG02–92ER61396.

Wilson, W.J. (1987) *The Truly Disadvantaged*. Chicago: University of Chicago Press.

Yantzi, N., Rosenberg, M.W., Burke, S.O. and Harrison, M.B. (2001) 'The impacts of distance to hospital on families with a child with a chronic condition', *Social Science and Medicine*, 52(12): 1777–1791.

Part III

Knowledge, governance and the future

Chapter 9

Public health and the 'new genetics'

Balancing individual and collective outcomes

Evan Willis

Introduction

The 'dawning' and 'heralding' metaphors have had a lot of use recently. They have been widely used as a new millennium has coincided almost exactly with a 'new age' of genetically based health care following the completion of the first draft of a map of the human genome about the middle of its first year. But if the 'dawning' metaphor has been a powerful one for the science of genetics, it has occurred under overcast conditions as far as the understanding of the social implications (including legal and ethical) of new and more powerful maps are concerned.

This chapter considers the consequences for one particular field of health care of these developments, namely public health. Rather than attempt to analyse these implications in general, three specific case studies are developed in this chapter. It considers the main social policy issue that arises as the project unfolds; one of maximizing any benefits that may arise and minimizing any drawbacks. If advances in the understanding of the genetic basis of disease have outpaced the related understanding of the social and societal implications, how can social scientists contribute to the evolution of policies to guide and regulate the new genetically based technologies, their development, practices and the uses to which they are put? Such policies are needed at all levels: individuals, families, societies and globally.

Public Health

Several caveats to the analysis should be mentioned first. While public health is conventionally defined in terms of the organized effort by society in disease prevention and health promotion, the term is commonly used in two senses: public in contrast to private health on one hand and public in contrast to clinical on the other. This chapter focuses on the latter; perhaps more academically based definition, being mainly concerned with the usage of the term public health in contrast to clinical medicine practised at the bedside. The difference between the two are ones of emphasis: on prevention rather than treatment, on providing the conditions under which disease can be minimized and health promoted through safe water, clean air, safe working conditions and so on (see Detels et al. 1997). Traditionally concerned with working and living conditions, and based upon the discipline of epidemiology, a 'new public health' has emerged with the Ottawa Charter and the Alma Ata declaration (Baum 1998).

Second, none of what is written below should be interpreted in such a way as to deny the individual burden of genetic disease. The focus of this chapter instead is about the balance between individual and collective uses of the knowledge arising from the new genetics and the technologies based upon that knowledge. Third, nor should the chapter read as emphasizing excessively the differences between geneticists on one hand and the public health community of academics and practitioners on the other (see Cunningham-Burnley and Kerr 1999). Both groups deal at the population level and study the interaction between genetic and environmental factors. The common ground between the two groups is substantial in other words with many geneticists acutely aware of the social, legal and ethical issues that flow from the Human Genome Project (HGP).

The opportunities

There is now a substantial literature on the opportunities that advances in genetic understanding of disease offers for the improvement of human health and that is not in contention here (see for example Bodmer and McKie 1997). There is also plenty written on how to maximize the benefits such advances may bring and the whole emerging discipline of public health genetics is dedicated to that end (see for example Khoury et al. 2000). What there is rather less of is a literature on how the 'new genetics' is affecting health policy (see Kaufert 2000; Petersen and Bunton 2002; Pilnick 2002). This chapter will focus instead on the challenges and indeed the dangers of these advances and how social scientists may contribute to the process of minimizing these.

The question is one of balance; maximizing the upside while acknowledging that a downside does exist and must be confronted with regulatory and other strategies. Balancing the positives with the negatives is a policy issue at a number of levels. This is especially in the context of the health and social policy issue of the appropriate role of genetic testing; studied among others by the US task force on genetic testing run as part of the ELSI aspect of the HGP (Holtzman and Watson 1997). Questions of insurance, employment, discrimination and loss of privacy together constitute potentially the downside of developments to be guarded against, alongside the benefits (see for example Otlowski 2001).

But it is the broader implications for public health with which this chapter deals. As Bunton and Petersen (2002: 96) argue, 'working concepts of the environment, the host and the agent in public health become destabilised when genetic technologies subject each to manipulation and choice'. There are a number of relevant issues but the concentration here is the classic tension between individual and collective uses of emerging genetic biotechnologies. These technologies do not occur in a vacuum but as part of a social context which must be taken into consideration. The genetic biotechnologies have both individual uses and collective uses and the potential exists for a tension to exist between the two.

Three case studies

The shape of the impact of the HGP on public health is only beginning to emerge. Furthermore, while there seem to be some common issues, it is difficult to discuss the impact in general terms. Instead three case studies will be briefly considered and then analysed.

Ozone and the melanoma gene

In 1997, the biotechnology firm Myriad genetics was awarded a patent on the MTS1 (Multiple Tumor Suppressor 1) melanoma gene, which gave it the right to develop a test for the identification of individuals who have an increased risk of developing melanoma through inherited susceptibility (http://www.myriad.com/pr/19970430.html). What public health role might such a test have?

> An MTS1 genetic test for melanoma has the important potential role of alerting individuals at high risk for skin cancer to take precautionary measures before the cancer develops and to have suspicious lesions removed, so that the risk of melanoma may be substantially reduced in these individuals.
>
> (http://www.oncolink.upenn.edu/cancernet/99/dec/712705.html#11)

So, at the individual level, high-risk individuals can be identified, monitored as well as counselled what they can do to reduce the likelihood of developing melanoma. Currently at both the individual level as well as the group level of melanoma-prone family members, management recommendations include monthly skin self-examination, clinical skin examination once or twice yearly, a low threshold for simple excision of changing pigmented lesions, moderation of sun exposure and appropriate use of sunscreens (Greene 1999).

What relevance would such tests have for the residents of the southern Chilean city of Punta Arenas of 120,000 residents, 3500 kilometres south of the Chilean capital of Santiago, when the hole in the ozone layer over Antarctica reached a world population centre for the first time in the spring of 2000, exposing residents to the very high levels of ultraviolet radiation that can cause melanomas and making the city 'ground zero' for the effects of climate change?

> Government authorities in Punta Arenas last week unveiled a special public education program urging citizens to take precautions from the fierce glare of ultraviolet radiation caused by the depleted ozone layer . . . The program – 'Magallanes Ozone 2000' – instructs citizens to minimize their exposure to the sun by wearing wide-brimmed hats, long pants and long sleeved shirts, and religiously apply sunscreen on a daily basis . . . Other program recommendations include keeping infants entirely out of the sun until six months of age. Older babies and children should only go in the sun for short periods of time and always with plenty of sunscreen . . . The yellow alert does not include suspending school classes but does mean that sports practices and other activities cannot be held out of doors.
>
> (http://oc.orientation.com/en/topstories/6731404.html)

Individualizing the risk of skin cancer by allocating resources to screening of course does have a place in responding to the risk. But arguably, in this case (perhaps the first of many such cases), individualist solutions are less important than collective responses. Everyone needs to follow precautionary measures at an individual level as well as pursue collective action. Collectivizing the risk of skin cancer would result in political agitation to encourage implementation of the 1987 Montreal Protocols to eliminate CFCs (chlorofluorocarbons) as well as the 1997 Kyoto Protocol to reduce greenhouse gas emissions that have led to ozone thinning, in the face of attempts by a US president beholden to greenhouse polluters for massive campaign contributions to abandon them, or at least water them down.

The social context is important further in influencing the societal response and deciding resource allocation in a developing country. On what health strategy should public health authorities spend a limited public health budget to deal with the citizens having become the subjects of a global environmental experiment of 'what are the consequences of living under the growing ozone hole?'

Patented gene testing technology to screen for those with heightened susceptibility does not come cheaply. Nor are city authorities keen to publicize the extent of the risk because of the threat to the city's attempts to build a tourism industry. Issuing health alerts that those with pale skin can stay in the sun for only seven minutes is hardly contributing to such an aim. Nor are the city's infamous high winds conducive to the erection of shade measures or even hats staying on. Not only that, but also the means of measuring ozone thinning as a basis for the issuing of alerts may not be available.

> Officials acknowledge the critical need to address the problem – but claim they won't be able to afford $180,000 for an ozone- and radiation-measuring instrument after Punta Arenas scientists return the only one they have later this month to the institute in Brazil from which they borrowed it.
>
> (MacKeen 2000)

Bladder cancer and chemical workers

The occupational health and safety of the workforce is one potential area of application of advances in the genetic understanding of disease. Here the balance of benefits and drawbacks depends on from whose point of view it is being considered. Bladder cancer in chemical industry workers is a classic case of an occupational health hazard (akin to chimney sweeps) and has long been documented, being one of the first workplace-induced cancers to be associated with industrialization (Kantoff et al. 1998). Systematic research as long ago as 1954 documented the relationship especially with a type of chemical known as aromatic amines (see Case et al. 1954).

The identification of the *p53* gene associated with bladder cancer (Semenza and Weasel 1997) has raised complex issues about the role of screening as part of pre-employment medical examinations. Should a putative test for mutations of the *p53* gene be given to workers and 'carriers' denied employment in the chemical industry? At the individual level, of course, it would appear prudent for the potential workers themselves to seek employment elsewhere rather than knowingly expose themselves to higher risk (though the salutary case is perhaps the 30% of the adult Australian population who smoke tobacco). At the collective level however the issues are a little different. Screening out potential workers compensation claimants among workers who subsequently develop bladder cancer is a means for chemical industry employers to use genetic biotechnologies for social control purposes to discriminate against those carrying the gene. Furthermore, the approach is compatible with the traditional method of dealing with occupational health and safety hazards summed up by the phrase 'fix the worker not the workplace'. If machinery is noisy, workers should wear hearing protection rather than quieter machinery being installed. Instead of discriminating against workers with the 'defective' gene, a more appropriate collective response (long favoured by trade unions) is to monitor the workplace to make it safer so harm to individual workers is minimized. As Draper (1996) argues:

> The important underlying question here is: Do we focus on the individual or on the environment? In fact, a certain percentage of people may develop these diseases and others may not, but in most cases the idea that a biological trait of the workers themselves causes the problem is unproven. Focusing on the individuals and their possible predispositions too often is a

> way of inappropriately changing the subject, away from the workplace hazards. Screening and monitoring are two major alternatives that have developed in response to the identification of genetic and biological traits and hazardous substances. Screening has developed as an alternative to monitoring, in that high-risk individuals have been identified and screened out as a favored means of reducing exposure to environmental contaminants. Employers increasingly favor a screening approach to environmental hazards. In fact, the screening approach is winning, which leads to some significant problems. The screening approach involves detecting individuals who then will be excluded from exposure to the toxic substance. In contrast, the declining monitoring approach involves monitoring contaminants in order to determine whether exposures are too high for those who are exposed to them – like measuring levels of air contaminants with a radiation badge.
>
> (Draper 1996)

Like genetic testing for inherited susceptibility to bladder cancer, testing for susceptibility to skin cancer represents the measuring of genetic risk within an individualist paradigm consistent with existing power structures of industry. In other words the social relations of the medical technology of genetic testing gives another more powerful social control tool for individualizing the risk of bladder cancer. An alternative approach, long favoured by unions, would be to work in eliminating cancer-causing agents from the workplace in general.

Haemochromatosis

There is a case where arguably individual and collective benefits coincide. Haemochromatosis (HH) is an

> autosomal recessive disease of iron regulation, resulting in excessive iron absorption and ultimately in iron overload, leading to end organ disease. Complications of HH include cirrhosis, primary liver cancer, cardiomyopathy, arthritis and diabetes. Screening studies using serum iron measures suggest a prevalence of 1/200–1/400 . . . In all clinical series, males outnumber females. HH is much rarer in Asians and African-Americans than in people of European descent. A different iron overload syndrome, probably genetic, has been described in African-Americans and sub-Saharan Africans. In 1996, a candidate gene for HH was identified adjacent to the major histocompatibility locus. The gene has been designated HFE . . . Removal of iron by phlebotomy increases survival in symptomatic patients. In a small cohort, institution of regular phlebotomy (3–4 times per year) prior to the development of cirrhosis or diabetes was associated with an apparently normal life expectancy.
>
> (Burke 1998)

So the complications of HH can be largely avoided by individuals donating blood three or four times a year, making it something of a model for evaluating the public health impact of genetics! Here an individual benefit potentially coincides with a public benefit. But whether the blood removed via phlebotomies can be entered into the blood supply is more problematic (as a specific treatment for iron deficiencies in others?). The Red Cross blood service in Australia recently decided to use it but it does not yet occur in the United States although there appear to be plans to do so as the 'stigma' associated with HH blood is removed (see http://www.victorherbert.com/ash1999.htm). It has not been utilized previously seemingly because of complications about the act of donating being both a chargeable treatment (for HH) and a money-earning act in the US system. There are also complexities about ensuring the safety of the blood supply by requesting information about sexual practices and the like, not usually a part of treatment regimes. The other model aspect of HH is its simplicity with (at least in the Australian context) commercial interest relatively absent.

But again, as trials of workplace screening of individuals for HH are planned in the Australian context (*The Age*, 18 October 2000), the question remains: should resources be spent identifying at-risk individuals to receive treatment for HH, or for encouraging greater levels of blood donation to ensure the blood supply for treatment purposes? The latter course of action also provides opportunities for screening of persons with HH at time of donation (see Khoury et al. 2000). Clearly the question is one of balance.

Individuals and the state

The tension between individual and collective interests is a common theme in the brief analysis of the case studies and can be considered more generally in the public health context. Some degree of regulation and restraint on the liberty of individuals is largely accepted in most societies in the promotion of public health although the extent varies societally. In the Australian context, quarantine, gun control, fluoridation of water supply and pasteurization of milk are examples, as are car seatbelt and bicycle helmet wearing and prohibition of mobile phone use while driving. How might discoveries in genetics be translated into public health action in this context? How can public health opportunities for health promotion and disease prevention be balanced against decisions concerning the appropriate use of information and technologies based upon these discoveries? In pursuing disease prevention and health promotion, balancing the rights of individuals against a state, pushed by rampant biotechnology commercial interests is a difficult health policy challenge for the future.

Most of the activity thus far has been of the mapping variety and actual technological innovations have been slower to follow. If gene therapy is still largely a feature of the predawn hopeful glow on the horizon of medicine then how else might these advances be translated into the full light of day?

The conventional distinction between primary, secondary and tertiary prevention is useful here although exactly how this scheme translates into the new genetics is far from clear. Primary prevention focuses on stopping the illnesses, genetic or otherwise, before they occur. Secondary prevention targets clinical manifestations of the disease by early detection, and tertiary prevention minimizes the effects of the disease by preventing complications and deterioration (see Khoury 1996: 1718).

Yet genetic testing technologies bring new questions to the issue of what it means to prevent or control disease. Applied to the field of genetic medicine, primary prevention involves prenatal testing and termination if the foetus is shown to carry the gene for particular conditions and likely to manifest that genetic illness during their lifetime. Yet social relations of prenatal diagnosis are complex. Not only are they tied up with the politics of abortion but also they involve the issue of the seriousness of the genetically caused disease. Clear eugenic overtones are implicit in the question of 'How perfect does a foetus, on the basis of prenatal diagnosis, have to be before the pregnancy is allowed to proceed to term?'

Secondary prevention involves and is being translated to mean genetic screening, such as for HH. Yet, as the case studies illustrate, the social relations of screening technology are complex. In recent history of medical technology assessment resolving issues of whether population screening for non-genetic conditions are safe, effective and cost-efficient have been muddied by a variety of factors not the least of which is an economic and commercial imperative that often masquerades as a technological imperative (see Willis 1997). The squabbling over the relative roles of commercial biotechnology company Celera Genomics vis-à-vis the publicly funded effort in the Human Genome Project (see Cook-Deegan 1994) does not augur well for resolving the complex health policy issues of whether to embark on genetic screening for a variety of genetically caused conditions that the new knowledge about the human genome has made possible.

Then there are difficulties in defining what is 'normal' and 'abnormal'; such definitions being both culturally and historically conditional. A Danish attempt to define what counts as a genetic disorder (i.e. to construct a list of diseases relevant for screening) was abandoned on the grounds that

> the question was not only medical but also social, and should be worked out in co-operation with patients. This question includes consideration of the implications of the following: degrees of severity of disorder (e.g., cleft lip vs. Huntington's disease) and variation within a disorder (e.g., mild vs. severe haemophilia), how the carrier state should be regarded, the importance of recognition of partial penetrance (the proportion of those with the genotype that manifest the phenotype), and the distinction between unifactorial and multifactorial conditions.
>
> (Chadwick et al. 1993)

The dangers

But if there are opportunities provided by the increase in the understanding of the genetic basis to disease, there are also many dangers. The remainder of this chapter analyses these. One is the overgenetization of disease. With a large increase in at least theoretical knowledge about particular conditions, a perhaps understandable frustration on the part of practitioners trying to assist their patients and an aggressive biotechnology industry keen to pursue the green fields of profitability from their inventions, a tendency has arisen to overemphasize the role of genetic factors. Cancer is a good example of overgenetization. It is widely accepted that the causes of cancer are a combination of genetic and environmental. Advances in genetic understanding of cancer have opened up new areas of research and treatment that it is hoped will help alleviate this scourge. Yet there is a tendency to overemphasize the genetic element in the manner described in the mid-1960s by Kaplan (1964: 64) as the Law of the Instrument: 'Give a small boy a hammer and he will find that everything he encounters needs pounding.' It echoes a Swedish saying that 'when you're holding a hammer everything looks like a nail'. In psychology, the phenomenon is called 'functional fixedness' or the Einstellung effect (Reiber 1995).

The new tools of genetic diagnosis and screening are in danger of being overemphasized; what's a genetic nail and what's not being confused. An example is breast cancer (see Hopper 1996). Emphasis on the 5–10% of cancers which are heritable has the potential to divert attention (and possibly research funding) from research on the 90–95% which are not and for which ongoing research on the environmental and other non-medical determinants remains crucial. As the Council for Responsible Genetics (1997) laments:

> The overemphasis on genetic factors in cancer, when environmental carcinogens are known to make major contributions, takes attention away from environmental cleanup measures that could, in fact, reduce the incidence of cancer. Current research has identified links between cancer and a host of non-genetic factors, including organochlorides, estrogen and estrogen-like chemicals, pesticides, radiation, bovine growth hormone, diet and exercise. The 'geneticisation' of cancer creates a blame-the-victim mindset that obscures these social and environmental factors.
>
> (Council for Responsible Genetics 1997)

Another danger that relates to the above is the tendency arising from greater genetic knowledge to individualize disease in a form of genetic reductionism; a sort of 'Genes 'R' Us' approach to the world. This fits neatly with an individualist paradigm of disease which views it as an individual and biological phenomenon which can be alleviated by direct procedures being carried out on individuals. Public health by contrast has tended to operate with a more social and political model of disease. Health can be promoted and disease reduced by collective action to secure clean water, shorter working hours, clean air, safe working environments. The new genetics has more than the potentiality to defuse and reduce the basis for collective action; it is already happening. Part of the attraction of the HGP has been that the better understanding of genetics fits neatly with a paradigm of economic and political orientation in which globalization and the dominance of the market have come to rule. Therefore if individuals get sick it is because of their genes rather than the environment in which they live or work. Remedial programmes can therefore be directed at those individuals rather than trying to improve the conditions of life and existence for everyone. Such a view fits neatly with the growing hegemony of American cultural values under globalization, where, as Nelkin and Lindee (1995) argue, the gene has become something of a cultural icon that

> intersects with important American cultural values. Genetic explanations appear to locate social problems within the individual rather than in society, conforming to the ideology of individualism. They are thus a convenient way to address troubling social issues; the threats implied by the changing roles of women, the perceived decline of the family, the problems of crime, the changes in the racial and ethnic structure of American society and the failure of welfare programs.
>
> (Nelkin and Lindee 1995: 194)

At the same time the emerging biotechnologies also provide a powerful instrument of social control through the bio-surveillance of populations permitting classification of individuals on the basis of genetic risk (for insurance as well as other purposes such as in the example of the occupational health and safety field detailed above) as well as a narrowing of the definition of what it means to be a 'normal' human being – information of considerable actuarial relevance.

Other dangers also arise out of the globalized nature of the HGP. The project is itself a force for globalization but the danger lies in the assumption that the social relations of the biotechnologies arising out of the project will be the uniform across the globe rather than reflecting particular historical and cultural contexts. Already these latter factors have been important. Germany was late to join the project reflective of the baggage of the Nazi era together with the eugenicist overtones of the HGP (see Cook-Deegan 1994). The first director of the HGP, James Watson, was asked how these abuses of the past could be avoided in the future with the project. His reported response was that the state should stay out of the picture since the abuses all occurred as official state policy (Wikler 2000).

Now apart from the problem that the 'state' is never conceptualized, this type of reported comment reflects a particularly North American concern where the politico-economic context historically and contemporarily has been to minimize the role of the state consistent with maximizing the opportunities for capital accumulation by the private sector. With such a cultural mindset then the suggested solution to past problems is for the state to have no role in the regulation of developing genetic biotechnologies and therefore presumably to allow market forces to determine the processes of invention, innovation and diffusion. The so-called 'technological imperative' turns out on closer examination to be an economic imperative, best pursued with minimal state intervention. In the Australian context, as in many other liberal democracies, the state has a history of intervention in public health to restrain market forces in the interests of not only legitimacy generally but also policy aims of equity (both of access and resource allocation). The United States indeed is unusual among Western liberal democracies in persisting with individual health including genetic risk management through private health insurance rather than community risk assumption through national health insurance schemes such as Medicare in Australia or the National Health Service in the United Kingdom. Restrictions on what Americans call the liberty of individuals in the interest of public health has long been accepted more in Australia and other countries than in the United States. So while Americans argue about whether the compulsory wearing of seatbelts interferes with one's god-given right to kill yourself in a motor accident, this public health measure has long been accepted in many other countries. Australians have supported the restrictions of guns in the community as a public health measure largely unencumbered with arguments about the 'right' to own and carry firearms. Similar examples are the compulsory wearing of bicycle helmets, the banning of the use of mobile phones while driving and many others. So the state is already heavily involved in the regulation of the knowledge arising from the improvements in public health and should continue to be so.

Another danger is the re-emergence of sociobiological explanations for human behaviour. Now broadly called evolutionary psychology, it is more sophisticated than some of the earlier controversial work (e.g. Wilson 1980). Advances in the genetic understanding of disease have generated interest in whether some sorts of behaviour can also be explained genetically. Those mentioned include various sorts of mental illness, homosexuality, alcoholism, obesity, homelessness and the Holy Grail of intelligence. But whereas in its earlier outbreak several decades ago, sociobiology pitched its explanation (for male dominance for instance) in terms of crude instinct and 'innateness', now evolutionary psychologists are able to go a step further in genetic reductionist explanation to explain human behaviour in genetic terms (see Dusek 1999). Fortunately the earlier critique of sociobiology has been expanded to include a powerful argument that individuals are not just the sum of their genes (see Rose et al. 1984; Rose and Rose 2000; David 2002) and that the relationship between nature and nurture remains a complex one in which both are relevant and important in explaining human behaviour. It is quite possible to acknowledge that all human diseases of public health importance are the result of the interaction between genetic variation and the environment, without resorting automatically to a genetic reductionist position of the pre-eminence of genetic causation.

The further danger however is the compatibility between this view of behaviour based upon evolutionary psychology and neo-conservative political agendas that now sweep the globe. Human societies are becoming increasing polarized into rich and poor, both globally and also relatively speaking within countries. A form of economic apartheid is emerging such that issues of social as well as environmental sustainability loom as social cohesion within and between countries is threatened. The dangers of explanations that locate the reasons for inequality in their crudest form in people's genetic make-up encourages and supports a political programme that sees inequality therefore as somehow natural and immutable. Interpreted in this way, the HGP provides a rationale and a justification for inequality. As a result state programmes to address the effects of inequality are not necessary or effective and cuts in government and aid spending that attempted to ameliorate this polarization legitimized by business elites. In that sense the globalizing nature and influence of the Human Genome Project has very much a negative aspect especially if the social relations of the biotechnologies that flow from the project have a strong flavour of American capitalism about them.

Conclusion

This chapter concentrates upon the broadest level of impact of advances in the genetic understanding to disease for public health in both its traditional and 'new' senses. The challenge, to which social scientists must be involved, is to harness the benefits of advances in the genetic understanding of disease and help ensure that these outweigh the apparent drawbacks. These drawbacks occur at several levels including that of commercial and other pressures including the tendency towards biosurveillance and social control. This chapter also points to a broader level; that of what might broadly be called the politico-economic context, to show the consequences (both intended and unintended) of the Human Genome Project on public health. Many of the policy decisions have to do with resource allocation questions of where to invest for maximum possible health gain. Crucial to this decision is the central social science issue of the relationship between the individual and society, or as expressed in health terms between individual and population health, in pursuing this aim.

Many questions remain that constitute a research agenda for social scientists. What might be the balance between individual and collective interests and how would one strike it? What might be some of the options before us and how might public debate be pursued in order to arrive at an informed community view? If gene technology was to be used expressly for public health benefit, what would be the applications and how would we know it?

To be clear, the argument here is not that amelioration of the individual manifestation of genetic disease should not be pursued. Instead it is argued that balancing resource allocation between individual and population health is a difficult task when the whole politico-economic context in which these advances are taking place is taken into consideration. Investment in population health issues is problematic as a result. The clear and present danger is that individual health ends are being sought at the expense of the sort of population health benefits that have always been the concern of public health.

References

Baum, F. (1998) *The New Public Health: An Australian Perspective*. South Melbourne: Oxford University Press.

Bodmer, W. and McKie, R. (1997) *The Book of Man: the Human Genome Project and the Quest to Discover our Genetic Heritage*. New York: Oxford University Press.

Bunton, R. and Petersen, A. (2002) 'Editorial: genetics, ethics and governance', *Critical Public Health*, 12(2): 95–101.

Burke, W. (1998) 'Hemochromatosis: public health implications of screening', Abstracts from the First Annual Conference on Genetics and Public Health. CDC Atlanta, http://www.cdc.gov./genetics/publications/abstracts.htm (accessed 21 November 2001).

Case, R., Hosker, M. and Macdonald, D. (1954) 'Tumours of the urinary bladder in workmen engaged in the manufacture and use of certain dyestuff intermediaries in the British chemical industry: part I', *British Journal of Industrial Medicine*, 11: 75–104.

Chadwick, R., Coli, D., ten Have, H., Husted, J., Pogliano, C. and Shickle, D. (1993) *A Report to the Commission of the European Communities: Ethical Implications of Human Genome Analysis for Clinical Practice in Medical Genetics with special reference to Genetic Counselling*. University of Wales, Cardiff Centre for Applied Ethics, http://www.uclan.ac.uk/facs/ethics/gencoun.htm (accessed 20 November 2001).

Cook-Deegan, R. (1994) *The Gene Wars: Science, Politics, and the Human Genome*. New York: Norton.

Council for Responsible Genetics (1997) *BRCA1 and Breast Cancer: Myths and Facts*. Boston, MA, http:www.essential.org/crg/BRCA-1.html (accessed 2 December 2001).

Cunningham-Burnley, S. and Kerr, A. (1999) 'Defining the "social": towards an understanding of the medical and scientific discourses on the social aspects of the "New Genetics"', *Sociology of Health and Illness*, 21(5): 647–668.

David, M. (2002) 'The sociological critique of evolutionary psychology: beyond mass modularity', *New Genetics and Society*, 21(3): 303–313.

Detels, R., Holland, W. and Knox, G. (1997) *Oxford Textbook of Public Health*, 3rd edn. New York: Oxford University Press.

Draper, E. (1996) 'Social issues of genome innovation and intellectual property', *Risk*, 7: 201–230, http://www.fplc.edu/risk/vol7/summer/draper.htm (accessed 29 October 2001).

Dusek, V. (1999) 'Sociobiology sanitized: the evolutionary psychology and genetic selectionism debates', *Science-as-Culture Forum*, http://www.human-nature.com/science-as-culture/dusek.html (accessed 19 November 2001).

Greene, M. (1999) 'The genetics of hereditary melanoma and nevi', *Cancer*, 86: 2464–2477.

Holtzman, N. and Watson, M. (1997) *Promoting Safe and Effective Genetic Testing in the United States*, Final Report of the Task Force on Genetic Testing. National Institutes of Health, Department of Energy Working Group on *Ethical, Legal, and Social Implications of Human Genome Research*, http://www.nhgri.nih.gov/ELSI/TFGT_final/ (accessed 24 November 2001).

Hopper, J. (1996) 'Some public health issues in the current state of genetic testing for breast cancer in Australia', *Australian and New Zealand Journal of Public Health*, 20(5): 467–472.

Hubbard, R. and Wald, E. (1999) *Exploding the Gene Myth*. Boston, MA: Beacon Press.

Kantoff, P., Anthony, L.. Zietman, A. and Wishnow, K. (1998) 'Bladder cancer', in J. Holland, E. Frei, R. Bast, D. Kufe, D. Morton and R. Weichselbaum (eds) *Cancer Medicine*, 4th edn. Chicago: Williams and Wilkins, http://intouch.cancer-network.com/CanMed/Ch125/125-2.htm (accessed 26 November 2001).

Kaplan, A. (1964) *The Conduct of Inquiry*. San Francisco, CA: Chandler.

Kaufert, P. (2000) 'Health policy and the "New Genetics"', *Social Science and Medicine*, 51(6): 821–829.

Khoury, M. (1996) 'From genes to public health: the applications of genetic technology in disease prevention', *American Journal of Public Health*, 86(12): 1717–1722.

Khoury, M., Burke, W. and Thomson, E. (2000) *Genetics and Public Health in the 21st Century: Using Genetic Information to Improve Health and Prevent Disease*. New York: Oxford University Press.

Kolberg, B. (2000) *Gene Therapy – Status and Prospects in Clinical Medicine*. SMM report 1/2000, Norwegian Center for Health Technology Assessment, http://www.oslo.sintef.no/smm/News/FramesetNews.htm (accessed 14 January 2005).

MacKeen, D. (2000) 'Life under the hole in the sky', http://www.salon.com/health/feature/2000/11/03/ozone/ (accessed 21 November 2001).

Nelkin, D. and Lindee, S. (1995) *The DNA Mystique: The Gene as a Cultural Icon*. New York: Freeman.

Otlowski, M. (2001) *Implications of Genetic Testing for Australian Insurance Law and Practice*, Occasional Paper no. 1. Hobart: Centre for Law and Genetics, University of Tasmania.

Petersen, A. and Bunton, R. (2002) *The New Genetics and the Public's Health*. London: Routledge.

Pilnick, A. (2002) *Genetics and Society: An Introduction*. Buckingham: Open University Press.

Reiber, A. (1995) *The Penguin Dictionary of Psychology*. Harmondsworth: Penguin.
Rose, H. and Rose, S. (eds) (2000) *Alas Poor Darwin: Arguments against Evolutionary Psychology*. London: Cape.
Rose, S., Lewontin, R. and Kamin, L. (1984) *Not in our Genes: Biology, Ideology and Human Nature*. Harmondsworth: Penguin.
Semenza, J. and Weasel, L. (1997) 'Molecular epidemiology in environmental health: the potential of tumor suppressor gene p53 as a biomarker', *Environmental Health Perspectives*, 105(1): 155–163.
Wikler, D. (2000) 'Should the state intervene in ethical decisions in genetics', *Proceedings Third Menzies Scholars Symposium Human Genome Research: How far should we go? The post genomic world*. Melbourne, October, http://home.vicnet.net.au/~menzies/ (accessed 21 November 2001).
Willis, E. (1997) The prostatic imperative and the social relations of medical technology, *International Journal of Technology Assessment in Health Care*, 13(4):602–12.
Wilson, E.O. (1980) *Sociobiology*. Cambridge, MA: Harvard University Press.
Wilson, J.M.G. and Jungner, G. (1968) *Principles and Practice of Screening for Disease*. Public Health paper. Geneva: WHO.

Chapter 10

More than code

From genetic reductionism to complex biological systems

Martha R. Herbert

Introduction

The discovery of the genetic code has touched off an explosion of biotechnology, much of it based on the notion that there exists a programme underlying life that can now be read and rewritten. The belief that scientists have decoded life's inner workings has aroused public enthusiasm and attracted venture capital. But properly understood, the results of genetics research have undermined the notion that genes are the key to organismic development and pathology. There is much – for example the realization that even 'single gene' disorders are influenced by multiple genes and by environment; the slow pace of associating genes with diseases; the failure of identification of 'disease genes' to lead to therapies; the poor predictive power of genetic tests; and technical problems with attempts at gene modification – to suggest that genes are inextricable from the complexity of biological systems and that living things are not reducible to genetic code. Although scientists and biotechnology corporations have fallen far short of fulfilling initial ambitions, their enormous investment of financial and intellectual capital dictates the ongoing pursuit of the genetic 'revolution'. But critical analysis of the record to date is now vital. Genetics can no longer be regarded uncritically as the key to all biological problems.

From early on, molecular genetics was framed in terms of a 'central dogma': DNA contains the master code dictating the composition of protein, RNA transcribes this master code and guides the construction of the proteins, and proteins do the work of cells and organisms (Crick 1958). DNA made the rules; everything else obeyed. Although this model has since served as a powerful filter on perception and experimentation, it is a great oversimplification. Meanwhile a large and complex biotechnological sector has developed, which still bases itself in important ways on conceptions of genetics that have been surpassed scientifically (Commoner 2002). The shortfalls of the industry and the science, and the problems they neglect, can be illuminated by a review of the developments that have undermined their constitutive assumptions. These developments, in turn, suggest alternative frameworks.

Code dreams

The notion of a genetic code was shaped by reductionism, with its assumption that there exist fundamental molecular units that determine the workings of all other aspects of living organisms. Long before the identification of DNA as code, genes were framed as the basic and governing units of life (Kay 1993; Keller 2000).

The emerging notion of information as digital complemented this genetic reductionism. The idea of a molecular genetic code dovetailed with the digital mentality of the emerging computer age. The notion that life could be understood most fundamentally not in terms of biochemistry, metabolism, form and substance, but rather as information, offered a tantalizingly simple release from the messy complications of the living world. All qualitative features of organisms seemed now in principle derivable from a code of information. Cracking the code of life became the prime task of biology.

The path from decoding to recoding seemed a logical next step. The capacity and will to technologize biology emerged at a time when capitalist economic growth required new frontiers for patentable innovation. Biotechnology promised boundless permutations, far more than the manipulations of the worlds of 'stuff' previously possible through organic chemistry, electrical engineering, etc. This biodigital combination suggested vast new bases for investment and development. The basis of this triumphalist exuberance is the expectation of a seamless path from naming traits to identifying their genes, and then to manipulating or transferring them. In the words of Robert Shapiro, Monsanto CEO:

> The historical model, the industrial-revolution model we live by now, says that our quality of life has to do with possession of things, of stuff. But it turns out that information doesn't occupy a lot of stuff and can create enormous value . . . Biotech is a subset of information technology. It's a way of encoding information in nucleic acids as opposed to encoding it in charged silicon. It's a way to create value without creating more stuff. I put a gene, which is information, into a cottonseed, and I don't have to spray stuff on the crop in order to control insects. That strategy strikes me as the right one for agriculture, just as it strikes me as the right one for post-industrial society.
>
> (quoted in Specter 2000).

The reduction of the physicality of DNA to notions of 'gene' and 'information' is biologically naive. Yet it pervades not only public relations but also regulatory policies and even many scientific research programmes. Nevertheless, the physical world does not smoothly validate this model. The accelerating march of molecular genetics research is not along a straight path to conclusive command and control of nature, but rather encounters surprises and considerable unanticipated complexity.

Genetic research undermines biodigital notions: variability, heterogeneity, complexity

With greater knowledge, the 'gene' concept has become more complex. No longer is it sufficient to explain cellular reproduction; instead we must pay attention to a larger set of networks (Keller 2000). 'One gene, one protein' has given way to recognition of alternative splicing, i.e. different segments of a single transcriptional unit are now seen to play a variable role in different cellular contexts (Ewing and Green 2000). The folding up of polypeptide chains has never yet been predicted from DNA sequence information alone; it is crucially mediated by 'chaperone' molecules, and it is sensitive to intracellular and extracellular factors that are not traceable to individual gene determination (Cohen 2000). Processing of proteins after they are sequenced by DNA (such as by glycosylation, which adds sugar groups to parts of the amino acid sequence and affects protein function) proceeds differently in different tissues and among various species (Riddihough and Pennisi 2001). Chromosome structure and DNA methylation (Gibbs 2003b) and not merely DNA base sequence, are involved in determining gene expression (Kass and Wolffe 1998; Jenuwein and Allis 2001). What was previously called 'junk DNA' now appears to have function, playing regulatory roles (Gibbs 2003a). And while genes have been identified that appear to participate intimately in the generation of an organism's form or function, inactivation of such genes, or even their complete removal from the germline, often has little or no effect on development (Sigmund 2000). The development of form itself is not fully explicable in genetic terms (Newman and Müller 2000). Embryos with identical genes can develop into morphologically distinct organisms if environmental conditions are different, e.g. control of whether certain reptiles are male or female depends on temperature (Deeming and Ferguson 1988) and control of vertebrate number in certain strains of mice depends on the uterine environment (McLaren and Michie 1958).

Notions of 'one gene, one disease (or one trait)' are also being undermined. Gene researchers have sought to unearth the 'genes for' physical and neuropsychiatric disease states, as well as for behavioural and social features ranging from intelligence and physical prowess to violence. Hitherto there has been no direct mapping from DNA to protein to such observable human behavioural traits or disorders, and even the notion of such simple mapping is inappropriate (Newman 1988b; Hubbard and Wald 1999; Paterson et al. 1999). It would indeed be peculiar if hundreds of millions of years of evolution led in a direct line to a chemical code that 'determined' human and animal behaviour in a manner unambiguously reflective of the hierarchical structures of capitalist industrial society. Notions of direct mapping from gene to behaviour are also dubious from the vantage point of cognitive neuroscience, since between genes, proteins and behaviour lie many mediating levels and processes, including not only social influences but also variations in brain and body biology that are not fully determined by genes. There will be no straight path from gene to behaviour through this web of intersecting influences.

The notion that there are 'genes for' schizophrenia, autism, depression and so forth has led to a search for such genes that has as yet produced no 'answers'. While genome-wide screens have identified likely genes, and candidate genes have been investigated, these findings have largely not been replicated. At present no 'genes for' behavioural traits or neurobehavioural disorders have been unambiguously identified. Indeed, Steven Hyman, former Director of the U.S. National Institute of Mental Health, says:

> Gone is the notion that there is a single gene that causes any mental disorder or determines any behavioral variant. The concept of the causative gene has been replaced by that of genetic complexity, in which multiple genes act in concert with non-genetic factors to produce a risk of mental disorder.
> (Hyman 2000)

Inadequacy of quantitative response to qualitative complexity

Many behavioural geneticists who have not come around to Hyman's perspective respond to the growing complexity of the relationship of gene and environment to behaviour by simply hunting for ever more genes. One may sympathize; reconciling the implications of a polygenic model that has environmental interactions with existing research programmes is indeed challenging (Wahlsten 1999; De Jong 2000). In so far as there is genetic vulnerability, it is likely to be modulated not by a single gene but by a much larger range of genes, whose alleles (or versions) vary widely in the general population. The genes involved will code for a network of proteins, whose interactions will be almost impossibly complex to model. Furthermore, individuals will have differing subsets of these genes, and while all who share a diagnosis will have some common behavioural features, underlying causes may vary. Moreover, the genes themselves may not 'code for' the disease itself with inevitability, but only set up a vulnerability that requires subsequent environmental interaction, sometimes called a 'second hit' (London 2000). When the relative impacts of gene, environment and gene–environment interaction are parcelled out by statistical analyses, the proportional impact of a 'gene' by itself is often relatively small (though one should note that this notion of 'parcelling out' these influences is itself an oversimplification). In autism and some other neurobehavioural disorders the picture is further complicated by statistics indicating that incidence may have sharply increased (Kaye et al. 2001; Blaxill 2004). Such an increase is consistent with more complex gene–environment models, but it plays havoc with simple genetic determinism.

Internal variability of disease and gene 'entities'

Diseases themselves are not unitary entities. Diseases that merely 'look alike' (i.e. have the same phenotype) do not necessarily have the same genetic features (i.e. genotype). In these cases, the entity is not one disease, but many diseases. Thus, a limiting factor in genetic research is selection of a homogeneous group of subjects (Nagel 1999; Gillberg and Coleman 2000). In neurobehavioural disorders, the defining behavioural criteria are especially imprecise and no reliable biological markers have yet been discerned; hence some researchers are abandoning diagnosis-based investigations and looking at intervening levels, for example trying to correlate genes with 'endophenotypes', which include cognitive processing abnormalities involving more definable neural systems features (Leboyer et al. 1998). Moreover, phenotypic and genotypic variability are not limited to the behavioural domain, but are ubiquitous in physical disease states as well. Although certain nucleic acid sequences are associated with certain heritable diseases, the steps between this association and a full explanation of how these sequences lead to what we see as the disease have not been accomplished.

Prior to its identification with DNA sequences, the term 'gene' often signified presumed 'unit factors' underlying inheritance (Kay 2000). When it was first characterized, DNA appeared to embody the chemical basis of these unit factors. However, this model clashes with the picture emerging from further research: first, individual genes are not unitary factors but complex entities with potential for significant internal variability; second, individual genes do not function by themselves but are virtually always modulated and regulated by other genes or other physiological pathways; third, what genes do in any case is to code for the composition of proteins which do the real work within living organisms; fourth, proteins virtually always act in complex systems of multiple proteins; and fifth, it is in principle impossible to predict fully the range of functions of proteins and their interactions from information about genes (Strohman 1993, 2000; Huang 2000).

In 'monogenic' disorders, whose inheritance is associated with a single gene, the mutant gene has been thought to predict the disease entity. A few thousand such 'monogenic' disorders have been identified, and many or most of them are quite rare. They are classically distinguished from 'polygenic' disorders, which make up the vast bulk of genetically modulated disease. The notion of polygenic disorder implies influence by multiple genes, as well as by environmental factors; no single factor may dominate. However, with further research we see that even monogenic disorders are complex entities with many influences, not just the primary gene abnormality (Scriver and Waters 1999; Weatherall 1999; Dipple and McCabe 2000). Contributing to this are the many ways a single gene may mutate, the variable modulating effects of other genes, and environmental effects on gene expression and organismic functioning.

In terms of DNA, a gene is a lengthy and often discontinuous sequence of nucleotides that can be altered, or mutated, at many different sites along its length as well as in a variety of fashions (e.g. deletions, substitutions, frameshifts). Thus, mutation is not digital; instead, a gene can be altered in many ways each of which may have a different effect. As a result, while gene alterations may change amino acid sequences in proteins, there is a huge spectrum of potential variations between proteins that function 'normally' and proteins that do not function at all: proteins are not digital in their viability. An extreme is that a gene may not be translatable into any protein at all, or into any protein that can serve a function. But mutations can change as well as remove function. For example, substituting one base for another may change an individual amino acid in a protein. This may change the number and distribution of electrical charges and other physical properties in the sequence of amino acids, and these changes could cause the protein to fold differently. Altered protein folding can alter protein function, because proteins act not as linear strings but as three-dimensional entities, where what is hidden inside and what is exposed make a difference. A structural protein thus altered may still do its job but less well; an enzyme thus altered may still catalyze its chemical reactions but do so much more slowly. Structural or enzymatic changes like these can create a chronic disease state or can put the affected organism at risk of being more easily overwhelmed if environmental factors make extra demands on that structure or chemical pathway. And such a spectrum of possible alterations can apply to every component of an interacting network. The potential complexity and variability is immense.

Context heterogeneity is intrinsic to disease manifestations

Heterogeneity in gene effects is related to external as well as internal context. The function of every gene can be modulated in multiple ways by other genes, and there is great variability in this modulation. In the well-known 'monogenic' disorder phenylketonuria (or PKU), variability in mutations, modulating genes and environmental factors all influence the character and severity of disease expression. There are around 400 different alleles (or versions) of the gene involved with PKU, most of which are implicated in some form of the disease. The alleles result in variations in quantity of enzyme synthesized, in enzyme activity, and in the rate at which the enzyme is degraded. These changes are a consequence not only of differences in the gene and the resulting protein but also of variation in the pathways in which the gene product participates. Even in individuals with the identical allele, these other pathways may differ significantly, and the genes modulating these other pathways are likely to segregate separately from the primary gene locus, so that non-identical siblings may inherit different sets of modulatory genes. Moreover, PKU disease expression is dependent on dietary exposure to phenylalanine, and even genetically identical individuals can differ in this environmental respect (Scriver and Waters 1999). In thalassaemia, a disease of the blood's haemoglobin, in addition to all of the above classes of variability a geographical–environmental modulation has been identified, relating to patterns of exposure to infection and even to climate (Weatherall 1999). Even sickle-cell anaemia, the first 'single gene' disease to have been characterized at the molecular level, has a wide range of disease manifestations depending on other physiological and genetic aspects of the affected individual's biology (Mozzarelli et al. 1987).

Carrying a gene thought to be associated with a disease may not lead to disease at all; conversely, the disease phenotype can be created by pathways not related to the gene. In haemochromatosis, while a significant portion of people with the 'gene for' haemochromatosis do not develop the disease, a cohort has been found with clinically classic disease who do not have the associated gene mutation (Olynyk et al. 1999; Pietrangelo et al. 1999). In the early 1960s Gruneberg, in a classic study, showed that mice with a variety of skeletal disorders originally identified as 'genetic' could be bred so that even though the progeny still carried the disease-linked genes, they no longer showed signs of the disorders (Grüneberg 1963).

In sum, the notion that the genetic code has digitalized biology gives way to ever more layers of complexity and variability. There is no simple correspondence between genotype and phenotype, between gene and trait. While molecular biology has opened up vast new realms for investigation, it has also given us new measures of the profound limitations of our knowledge. As Craig Venter said after his corporation sequenced the human genome: 'We don't know shit about biology' (quoted in Preston 2000).

Biological complexity and critiques of geneticization

Our increasing appreciation of the complexity of biology and of the humbler, non-determinative role of genes in relation to larger organismic and ecological systems raises a number of questions that need to be addressed critically. The first is evaluating the extent to which the productivity of genetic research and of the biotech industry has been held back by their adherence to oversimplified models (Gilbert and Sarkar 2000). The second is evaluating the discrepancies between industry claims and the usually more limited actual capabilities in genetically related interventions already under way. The third is assessing the pressures driving competing reformulations of genetic and biological discourses in the light of this complexity that can no longer be ignored. Economic pressures to maintain a theory about the nature of genes and organisms that is compatible with ongoing investment and production may conflict with growing knowledge about complexity and interconnectedness. The roads taken and not taken by biological technologies will be affected by the outcome of these conflicts, as will the problems acknowledged or ignored, and solved or created.

Impact of models on productivity

Many public claims of the biotechnology industry have rested on notions of gene function and manipulability that are increasingly outdated. Certainly the hype produced to generate venture capital for this industry has conveyed assumptions about genetics that are strikingly more simplified that what is emerging from research (Petersen 2001). Arguments to restrict regulatory interference, in their minimization of risk, also brush aside complexity. Many public statements by involved scientists are in the same vein. A perusal of the industry's enterprises also conveys that their underlying philosophy has not fully anticipated the complexities encountered. It is thus not surprising that the industry has in fact encountered substantial resistance from complex organisms that resist its attempts at manipulating them on the basis of simpler gene-based models. This resistance has had fiscal consequences: on account of uncooperative organisms, many enterprises have not been able to fulfil their promises to investors.

This resistance has occurred in a number of sectors. Overall, various observers have noted that in medicine the impact of genetics to date on therapies has been limited (Holtzman and Marteau 2000; Le Fanu 2000). A striking failure has been the attempt to apply genetic knowledge therapeutically through *in vivo* genetic intervention. Gene therapy for severe combined immunodeficiency appeared to be an exception (Cavazzana-Calvo et al. 2000), but two patients subsequently developed leukaemia related to the treatment (Chinen and Puck 2004); there have thus been no successful somatic gene therapies to date (Lamb et al. 2000; Rosenberg and Schechter 2000; Saltus 2000). Gene therapy failures have arisen from multiple causes, including but not limited to genetic variability and to the influences from other factors discussed above that gene therapy does not address. Ignorance of the role of complex physiological networks in which the gene participates has stymied trials, yet analysis of gene therapy failures has not aroused great curiosity about analysing the role of these networks. In addition, there have been failures and even deaths due to immune rejection of the viral vector required to get the therapeutic gene agent into the patient. Thus, genes have not provided direct 'surgically precise' entry into targeted manipulation of the human organism. More recently, the gene therapy sector has been shifting its rhetoric toward plans to address more common diseases with more complex genetic models (Martin 1999). In truth, though, this new rhetoric will not alter the basically random character of gene therapy manipulations nor diminish the associated risks. It is thus doubtful that current biological and informatics approaches to complexity will be sufficient to secure the co-operation of the organism with the enterprise.

In other sectors, complexity has also dampened initial exuberance. For the pharmaceutical industry, genetics has been an aid but not a means of decoding all obscurity. While pharmacogenomics, through an integration of high-speed processing techniques with bioinformatics (Howard 2000), offers the allure of streamlined drug development, these techniques are not applicable across the board. They may slow as well as speed the process, thus sometimes increasing rather than decreasing drug development costs. For example, rapid screening of the genome may produce a glut of potential targets, many of which will be hard to assess; and computer ('in silico') modelling of chemical processes is currently applicable to only a minority of drug targets. Moreover, that human beings seem to have not much more than 30,000 genes further confirms that genes and proteins are likely to play numbers of roles in multiple bodily systems, so that drugs developed in the laboratory out of context of the organism will still need to be assessed in living human beings for unexpected detrimental effects, at significant unavoidable expense. Clinical trials, however, are a frustrating bottleneck with heavy pressures for ethical compromises, including conflicts of interest, more lax standards in privately funded research, and highly questionable practices in countries without regulations or enforcement power (Stephens et al. 2000).

Claims versus capabilities

Screening and surveillance may not be greatly enhanced by new types of genetic testing and profiling. The sequenced human genome will certainly yield more tests for disease-associated alleles. But while markets for these genetic applications may proliferate, the actual impact on health will probably be considerably less than one would expect for all the activity (Holtzman and Marteau 2000). For a small number of diseases, genetic tests are fairly predictive. For many others the predictive power is poor, leaving people painfully juggling probabilities. And even where predictive power is strong, such as in Huntington's disease, the test is often avoided (Hersch et al. 1994). The pharmaceutical industry's hope that drug-related genetic profiling will allow more systematic choice of subjects for drug trials and more rational prescription of drugs will probably be frustrated by the nonlinear properties of the genotype–phenotype relationship, which will always make predictions about individual response to new drugs uncertain. Thus, profiling will identify some people with extreme vulnerabilities, but for most people it is not likely to yield decisive information. Moreover, characterization of genetic risk of a small number can be accomplished only by genotyping of large populations, creating risk of genetic discrimination and surveillance (Nelkin and Andrews 1999). But projects of frankly predictive population surveillance will be dogged by the dubious relationship of genes with behavioural traits (Newman 1988a; Hyman 2000). The prospects of having anything like a comprehensive profile of genes predisposing to socially undesirable behaviours is remote, so attempts to sort and stigmatize people with such genetic tests will not sort people according to the intended divisions. Because of this, examination of the social and marketing apparatus for delivering and legitimizing all of these genetic testing applications will need to be informed by a sensitivity not only to social control and eugenics, but also to discrepancies between promises of precision and weak or erroneous performance deriving from inherent limitations to what identification of genes can predict.

Controversies about stem cell research also raise issues about whether promises are backed up by research. Twenty years of embryo stem cell research in mice has generated few, and modest, therapeutic effects in models of human diseases (Newman 2001). Moreover, it is concerning that embryonic stem cells are interesting to cancer researchers because they express genes not active in mature organisms except in tumours (Monk and Holding 2001), and because they have known tendencies to produce tumours (Martin 1981; Smith 2001a) as well as anatomical and physiological anomalies that may be hard to control in therapeutic applications. The reasons why adult stem cells – which have demonstrated efficacy and would not pose these safety problems or other ethical problems – have nevertheless been far less attractive deserves careful study. The developmental instabilities associated with embryonic stem cells also underly fundamental objections to human cloning and germline manipulation (Billings et al. 1999; Wunder 1999, 2000; Humphreys et al. 2001). Advocates of such techniques who aim for 'human enhancement' (Stock and Campbell 2000) or even outright transcendence of human species limitations (More 1999) assume that adequate technical control is imminent. They do not assimilate the implications of the participation of genes in multiple regulatory networks, nor the role of non-DNA in gene regulation, and how these preclude foreknowledge of what complications – including cancers, immune diseases and other developmental anomalies – might ensue from germline manipulations (Newman and Raffensperger 2000). Thus, claims for imminent disease cures or designer babies are overstated, to say the least.

Competing shifts to genetic complexity

As genetic complexity, as well as the shortfalls of genetics products as compared to what was promised enter more widespread awareness, leading figures in genetics research communities are making new admissions regarding the limitations of the field (Preston 2000; Collins et al. 2001), though sometimes claiming disingenuously that they had understood this complexity all along (Anonymous 2002). For example, within weeks of the announcement of the sequencing of the human genome, the horizon was shifted from genomics to proteomics and metabolomics, i.e. the description of the complement of proteins and metabolic products produced by an organism. There is more talk of going beyond genes to gene–environment interactions. But while gene language has shifted from determination to risk and complexity, such shifts in language can give a misleading appearance of advancing critical thinking that masks a failure to genuinely respond to the problems (Huang 2000; Haag and Kaupenjohann 2001). Rhetoric shifts faster than research agendas. More worrisome regarding risk, industry's 'sound science' regulatory approach is still remote from the 'precautionary principle' approach. Yet precaution is arguably more appropriate, since the uncertainty that goes hand-in-hand with complexity needs to be anticipated with active concern (Kriebel et al. 2001; Van Den Belt and Gremmen 2002).

In particular, the newer discourses that claim orientation to complexity may still collude in a problematic privileging of genetics in relation to the rest of biology. Such a privileging may occur out of an active assumption that all of biology is derivable from genes, but it may also occur passively, by default, out of relative ignorance of other relevant levels of biological investigation and functioning deriving from a lopsided focus in education and media (Nelkin and Lindee 1995). The many steps that lie between genes and organism functioning or ecological interactions, if not ignored, are often signified by terms like 'environment' or 'social influences' without being spelled out genetics then becomes implicitly equated with biology and also with determination. Genetics thus becomes a place-holder, a proxy, for the much broader universe of biology (Haila and Taylor 2001). But in actual practice, there are many instances where genetics is just a moment in a more complex set of inquiries involving non-genetic parts of biology. Certainly the great majority of effective medical treatments do not involve a clear understanding of the genetic component of the intervention, and were arrived at through astute observations at other levels than genetics. This is not to deny that genetics as a research tool can make strategic contributions in clarifying the nature of normal and maladaptive physiological processes. Physiological understanding can be refined through genetic investigations, whose results can be further clarified through more physiological study. Still, rather than being thought of as supplanting organismic biology and serving as the ultimate key to the nature of disease, genetics can be alternatively framed as just one stage in a complex physiological (and/or, depending on the questions, developmental, ecological or evolutionary) research programme. In medicine, therapies emerging from such programmes may target physiological processes only loosely linked to particular genes, even though the genes may have helped to identify the target processes. In many cases a gene-associated metabolic problem can be addressed physiologically or even nutritionally rather than genetically; for example, at the same time as we witness the virtual lack of any successful gene therapy, upwards of fifty genetic diseases (particularly ones where a slow enzyme is involved) respond favourably to various nutritional therapies (Elson-Schwab et al. 2002).

A social and public health rather than reductionist or commercial framing of complexity would situate genetics in the setting of biology including ecology, and also in the setting of culture, society and economies. Pivotal research domains here are the environmental genome project and toxicogenetics (National Institute of Environmental Health Sciences (NIEHS) 1999; Smith 2001b). In their study of genes relevant to the body's responses to toxic substances, they reveal that while individuals have genetically varying vulnerability they also face non-inevitable (and shared) exposures. At a practical level this broader framing of genetics in explicit relation to the environment expands the range of somatic information that can contribute to reflexivity in individual risk assessment, choices and responsibility (Novas and Rose 2000). Indeed, tests for non-genetic somatic information, such as for nutritional status, toxicant exposure and detoxification capacities – all centrally related to the 'second hits' that can turn genetic risk into disease (Ames 2001) – are within the horizon of science at its current level, and are sought by various communities because the information such tests can generate may have clearer implications for personal and social decision-making (Davis et al. 1998; Stein et al. 2002). Such non-genetic tests are subordinate in a commercial framework, not only because they are generally not patentable and less profitable, but also because their results can raise uncomfortable questions about environmental influences that call for social and public and not just personal and private remediation (Warhurst 2000). Thus, after getting test results listing one's own metabolic problems and burden of toxic chemicals, one may take measures as an individual to avoid toxic exposures, correct nutrient deficiencies, learn to exercise and relax more, and strengthen one's detoxification pathways (Parke 1991); but one may also join social movements working toward changing agricultural practices that nutritionally deplete food (Altieri 2000), as well as toward reducing job stress, stopping toxic emissions and developing sustainable agriculture and industry (Collins 2001; Geiser and Commoner 2001). The potential for such reflexive personal, public health and social interventions may be dampened by a gene-dominated perspective (Kerr and Cunningham-Burley 2000), but can be rekindled by locating somatic experience in a framework that is more broadly biological, which subsumes genetics in a larger context (Calver 2000; Montague and Pellerano 2001). This contextualizing of genetics is an important prerequisite to collective recognition of the shared risks created by industrial practices (Beck 1999).

Conclusion: genetics in a larger context

The problems faced by gene technologies suggest that organisms, like political subjects, are not so easily manipulated. Organisms will resist scientific theories that rationalize such manipulation, by acting in ways not predicted by the theories. This resistance underlies the poor performance of many domains of biotechnology. Sometimes problems deriving from complexity and unintended effects can be deferred until after a product is marketed. If the organism's resistance does not manifest itself until after a product is sold, the sector manufacturing it will do better (mainly due to lack of industry accountability) than if the resistance interferes with product development itself. But the recalcitrance of the organism will persist even as the boundaries of technical feasibility shift. Some theorists of biotechnology seem to take its promises at face value, and believe notions of interchangeability of genes and organismic components. This kind of theorizing blurs disjunctures between the intoxicating promises on the one hand and the actual outcomes – which may range from lacklustre to deeply disturbing. But rather than obscuring them, critical research programmes need to seek out these disjunctures, and the recalcitrance of organisms, and engage them explicitly and soberly.

The dominance of gene thinking in biology has been driven both intellectually and economically: reductionist models posit that genes ultimately determine all other levels of biological reality, and the biotechnology industry is based upon the commodifiability of genes. However, molecular genetics continually encounters problems that can be addressed only by looking beyond genetics. And commercialization of life favours patentable approaches, while many of the most pressing biologically related problems are insoluble by biotechnological interventions. The genetics and biotechnological enterprises are proceeding, but what can be investigated or produced is strongly technically constrained. There are economic imperatives to recruit these constrained technical capacities, whether or not what they produce has relevance for health and environmental considerations. Meanwhile, many other approaches have advantages in practicality, safety and sustainability, though perhaps not profitability. This leads to contention around allocating resources to non-genetic but biologically intelligent alternatives, as well as around the framing of discourses about complexity and gene–environment interactions. Critics and social movements argue that the 'geneticization' of biology and of society has meant a voracious and manic consumption of public resources for an enterprise that may continue to produce much less than promised and divert unfairly from many other pressing challenges. The growing revelations of organismic complexity may reveal this geneticization to be in many ways a compulsion, which can perhaps be calmed if social pressures can effect an appreciation of biology more broadly understood, and of its relationships with cultures and economies (Taylor and Haila 2001).

References

Altieri, M. (2000) *Agroecology in Action*, http://www.cnr.berkeley.edu/~agroeco3/ (accessed 25 October 2004).

Ames, B.N. (2001) 'DNA damage from micronutrient deficiencies is likely to be a major cause of cancer', *Mutation Research*, 475(1–2): 7–20.

Anonymous (2002) 'Wag the dogma' (editorial), *Nature Genetics*, 30(4): 343–344.

Beck, U. (1999) *World Risk Society*. Cambridge: Policy Press.

Billings, P.R., Hubbard, R. and Newman, S.A. (1999) 'Human germline gene modification: a dissent', *Lancet*, 353: 1873–1875.

Blaxill, M. (2004) 'What's going on: the question of time trends in autism', *Public Health Reports*, 119(6): 536–551.

Calver, M.C. (2000) 'Lessons from preventive medicine for the precautionary principle and ecosystem health', *Ecosystem Health*, 6(2): 99–107.

Cavazzana-Calvo, M., Hacein-Bey, S., Yates, F., de Villartay, J.P., Le Deist, F. and Fischer, A. (2000) 'Gene therapy of human severe combined immunodeficiency (SCID)-X1 disease', *Science*, 288: 669–672.

Chinen, J. and Puck, J.M. (2004) 'Successes and risks of gene therapy in primary immunodeficiencies', *Journal of Allergy and Clinical Immunology*, 113(4): 595–603; quiz 604.

Cohen, F.E. (2000) 'Prions, peptides and protein misfolding', *Molecular Medicine Today*, 6: 292–293.

Collins, F.S., Weiss, L. and Hudson, K. (2001) 'Heredity and humanity: have no fear. Genes aren't everything', *The New Republic*, http://www.tnr.com (accessed 25 October 2004).

Collins, T. (2001) 'Toward sustainable chemistry', *Science*, 291: 48–49.

Commoner, B. (2002) 'Unraveling the DNA myth: the spurious foundation of genetic engineering', *Harper's*, 304(1821): 39–47.

Crick, F.H.C. (1958) 'On protein synthesis', *Symp. Soc. Exp. Biol.,* 12: 139–163.

Davis, D.L., Axelrod, D., Bailey, L., Gaynor, M. and Sasco, A.J. (1998) 'Rethinking breast cancer risk and the environment: the case for the precautionary principle', *Environmental Health Perspectives*, 106(9): 523–529.

De Jong, H.L. (2000) 'Genetic determinism – how not to interpret behavioral genetics', *Theory and Psychology*, 10(5): 615–637.

Deeming, D.C. and Ferguson, M.W. (1988) 'Environmental regulation of sex determination in reptiles', *Philosophical Transactions of the Royal Society: Biological Sciences*, 322: 19–39.

Dipple, K.M. and McCabe, E.R.B. (2000) 'Modifier genes convert "Simple Mendelian Disorders" to complex traits', *Molecular Genetics and Metabolism*, 71: 43–50.

Elson-Schwab, I., Poedjosoedarmo, K. and Ames, B.N. (2002) KmMutants.org, http://www.KmMutants.org (accessed 25 October 2004).

Ewing, B. and Green, P. (2000) 'Analysis of expressed sequence tags indicates 35,000 human genes.' *Nature Genetics*, 25: 232–234.

Geiser, K. and Commoner, B. (2001) *Materials Matter: Toward a Sustainable Materials Policy (Urban and Industrial Environments)*. Cambridge, MA: MIT Press.

Gibbs, W.W. (2003a) 'The unseen genome: gems among the junk', *Scientific American*, 289(5): 46–53.

Gibbs, W.W. (2003b) 'The unseen genome: beyond DNA', *Scientific American*, 289(6): 106–113.

Gilbert, S.F. and Sarkar, S. (2000) 'Embracing complexity: organicism for the 21st century', *Developmental Dynamics*, 219(1): 1–9.

Gillberg, C., Coleman, M. (2000) *The Biology of the Autistic Spectrums (Clinics in Developmental Medicine)* 3rd edn. Cambridge: Cambridge University Press.

Grüneberg, H. (1963) *The Pathology of Development: A Study of Inherited Skeletal Disorders in Animals.* New York: Wiley.

Haag, D. and Kaupenjohann, M. (2001) 'Parameters, prediction, post-normal science and the precautionary principle – a roadmap for modelling for decision-making', *Ecological Modelling*, 144(1): 45–60.

Haila, Y. and Taylor, P. (2001) 'The philosophical dullness of classical ecology, and a Levinsian alternative', *Biology and Philosophy*, 16(1): 93–102.

Hersch, S., Jones, R., Koroshetz, W. and Quaid, K. (1994) 'The neurogenetics genie: testing for the Huntington's disease mutation', *Neurology*, 44(8): 1369–1373.

Holtzman, N.A. and Marteau, T.M. (2000) 'Will genetics revolutionize medicine?', *New England Journal of Medicine*, 343(2): 141–144.

Howard, K. (2000) 'The bioinformatics gold rush', *Scientific American*, 283(1): 58–63.

Huang, S. (2000) 'The practical problems of post-genomic biology', *Nature Biotechnology*, 18: 471–472.

Hubbard, R. and Wald, E. (1999) *Exploding the Gene Myth.* Boston, MA: Beacon Press.

Humphreys, D., Eggan, K., Akutsu, H., Hochedlinger, K., Rideout, W.M. 3rd, Biniszkiewicz, D., Yanagimachi, R., Jaenisch, R. (2001) 'Epigenetic instability in ES Cells and Cloned Mice', *Science*, 293(5527): 95–97.

Hyman, S.E. (2000). 'The genetics of mental illness: implications for practice', *Bulletin of the World Health Organization*, 78(4): 455–463.

Jenuwein, T. and Allis, C.D. (2001) 'Translating the Histone Code', *Science*, 293(5532): 1074.

Kass, S.U. and Wolffe, A.P. (1998) 'DNA methylation, nucleosomes and the inheritance of chromatin structure and function', *Novartis Foundation Symposium*, 214: 22–35.

Kay, L. (1993) *The Molecular Mission of Life: Caltech, The Rockefeller Foundation, and the Rise of New Biology.* New York: Oxford University Press.

Kay, L. (2000) *Who Wrote the Book of Life?* Stanford, CA: Stanford University Press.

Kaye, J.A., del Mar Melero-Montes, M. and Jick, H. (2001) 'Mumps, measles, and rubella vaccine and the incidence of autism recorded by general practitioners: a time trend analysis', *British Medical Journal*, 322(7284): 460–463.

Keller, E.F. (2000) *The Century of the Gene.* Harvard: Harvard University Press.

Kerr, A. and Cunningham-Burley, S. (2000) 'On ambivalence and risk: reflexive modernity and the new human genetics', *Sociology*, 34(2): 283–304.

Kriebel, D., Tickner, J., Epstein, P., Lemons, J., Levins, R., Loechler, E.L., Quinn, M., Rudel, R., Schettler, T., Stoto, M. (2001) 'The precautionary principle in environmental science', *Environmental Health Perspectives*, 109(9): 871–876.

Lamb, J.A., Moore, J., Bailey, A. and Monaco, A.P. (2000) 'Autism: recent molecular genetic advances', *Human Molecular Genetics*, 9(6): 861–868.

Leboyer, M., Bellivier, F., Nosten-Bertrand, M., Jouvent, R., Pauls, D. and Mallet, J. (1998) 'Psychiatric genetics: search for phenotypes', *Trends in Neuroscience*, 21(3): 102–105.

Le Fanu, J. (2000) *The Rise and Fall of Modern Medicine.* New York: Carroll and Graf.

London, E.A. (2000) 'The environment as an etiologic factor in autism: a new direction for research', *Environmental Health Perspectives*, 108(Suppl. 3): 401–404.

McLaren, A. and Michie, D. (1958) 'An effect of the uterine environment upon skeletal morphology in the mouse', *Nature*, 181: 1147–1148.

Martin, G.R. (1981) 'Isolation of a pluripotent cell line from early mouse embryos cultured in medium conditioned by teratocarcinoma stem cells', *Proceedings of the National Academy of Science USA*, 78(12): 7634–7638.

Martin, P. (1999) 'Genes as drugs: the social shaping of gene therapy and the reconstruction of genetic disease', in P. Conrad and J. Gabe (eds) *Sociological Perspectives on the New Genetics*. Oxford: Blackwell.

Monk, M. and Holding, C. (2001) 'Human embryonic genes re-expressed in cancer cells', *Oncogene*, 20(56): 8085–8091.

Montague, P. and Pellerano, M.B. (2001) 'Toxicology and environmental digital resources from and for citizen groups', *Toxicology*, 157(1–2): 77–88.

More, M. (1999) *The Extropian Principles, Version 3.0: A Transhumanist Declaration*, http://www.extropy.org/extprn3.htm (accessed 25 October 2004).

Mozzarelli, A., Hofrichter, J. and Eaton, W.A. (1987) 'Delay time of hemoglobin S polymerization prevents most cells from sickling in vivo', *Science*, 237: 500–506.

Nagel, R.L. (1999) 'Will the genetic individualization of disease force a new paradigm?' *Canadian Royal Academy of Science III*, 322(1): 1–4.

National Institute of Environmental Health Sciences (NIEHS) (1999) Environmental Genome Project, http://www.niehs.nih.gov/envgenom/concept.htm (accessed 30 October 2004).

Nelkin, D. and Andrews, L. (1999) 'DNA identification and surveillance creep', in P. Conrad and J. Gabe (eds) *Sociological Perspectives on the New Genetics*. Oxford: Blackwell.

Nelkin, D. and Lindee, S. (1995) *The DNA Mystique: The Gene as a Cultural Icon*. New York: WH Freeman.

Newman, S.A. (1988a) 'Does human genetic engineering have a scientific basis?', *Report from the Center for Philosophy and Public Policy*, 8: 6–9.

Newman, S.A. (1988b) 'Idealist biology', *Perspectives in Biology and Medicine*, 31: 353–368.

Newman, S. (2001) 'Embryo stem cells and biobusiness at 20', *GeneWatch*, 14(6): 5–6, http://www.gene-watch.org/ (accessed 25 October 2004).

Newman, S.A. and Muller, G.B. (2000) 'Epigenetic mechanisms of character origination', *Journal of Experimental Zoology*, 288(4): 304–317.

Newman, S. and Raffensperger, C. (2000) 'Genetic manipulation and the precautionary principle', in P.A. Norton and L.F. Steel (eds) *Gene Transfer Methods: Introducing Genes into Living Cells and Organisms*. Natick, MA: BioTechniques Books.

Novas, C. and Rose, N. (2000) 'Genetic risk and the birth of the somatic individual', *Economy and Society*, 29(4): 485–513.

Olynyk, J.K., Cullen, D.J., Aquilia, S., Rossi, E., Summerville, L. and Powell, L.W. (1999) 'A population-based study of the clinical expression of the hemochromatosis gene', *New England Journal of Medicine*, 341(10): 718–724.

Parke, D.V. (1991) 'Nutritional requirements for detoxication of environmental chemicals', *Food Additives and Contamination*, 8(3): 381–396.

Paterson, S.J., Brown, J.H., Gsodl, M.K., Johnson, M.H. and Karmiloff-Smith, A.

(1999) 'Cognitive modularity and genetic disorders', *Science*, 286(5448): 2355–2358.

Petersen, A. (2001) 'Biofantasies: genetics and medicine in the print news media', *Social Science & Medicine*, 52: 1255–1268.

Pietrangelo, A., Montosi, G., Totaro, A., Garuti, C., Conte, D., Cassanelli, S., Fraquelli, M., Sardini, C., Vasta, F., Gasparini, P. (1999) 'Hereditary hemochromatosis in adults without pathogenic mutations in the hemochromatosis gene', *New England Journal of Medicine*, 341(10): 725–732.

Preston, R. (2000) 'The genome warrior', *The New Yorker*, 66, June 12.

Riddihough G. and Pennisi E. (2001) 'The evolution of epigenetics', *Science*, 293(5532): 1063.

Rosenberg, L.E. and Schechter, A.N. (2000) 'Gene therapist, heal thyself' (editorial), *Science*, 287(5459): 1751.

Saltus, R. (2000) 'After bad gene found, no quick leap to a cure', *Boston Globe*, A01, Aug 7.

Scriver, C.R. and Waters, P.J. (1999) 'Monogenic traits are not simple: lessons from phenylketonuria', *Trends in Genetics*, 15(7): 267–272.

Sigmund, C.D. (2000) 'Viewpoint: are studies in genetically altered mice out of control?', *Arteriosclerosis, Thrombosis and Vascular Biology*, 20: 1425–1429.

Smith, A.G. (2001a) 'Embryo-derived stem cells: of mice and men', *Annual Review of Cell and Developmental Biology*, 17: 435–462.

Smith, L.L. (2001b) 'Key challenges for toxicologists in the 21st century', *Trends in Pharmacological Sciences*, 22(6): 281–285.

Specter, M. (2000) 'The Pharmageddon Riddle', *The New Yorker*, 58–71, Apr 10.

Stein, J., Schettler, T., Wallinga, D. and Valenti, M. (2002) 'In harm's way: toxic threats to child development', *Journal of Deveopmental and Behavioral Pediatrics*, 23(1 Suppl): S13–22.

Stephens, J., Flaherty, M.P, Nelson, D., LaFlaniere, S., Pomfret, J., DeYoung, K., Struck, D. (2000) 'The body hunters: international clinical drug testing', *Washington Post*, Dec 17.

Stock, G. and Campbell, J. (2000) *Engineering the Human Germline: An Exploration of the Science and Ethics of Altering the Genes we Pass to our Children*. Oxford: Oxford University Press.

Strohman, R.C. (1993) 'Ancient genomes, wise bodies, unhealthy people: limits of a genetic paradigm in biology and medicine', *Perspectives in Biology and Medicine*, 37: 112–145.

Strohman, R.C. (2000) 'Organization becomes cause in the matter', *Nature Biotechnology*, 18: 575–576.

Taylor, P. and Haila, Y. (2001) 'Situatedness and problematic boundaries: conceptualizing life's complex ecological context', *Biology and Philosophy*, 16(4): 521–532.

Van Den Belt, H. and Gremmen, B. (2002) 'Between precautionary principle and "sound science": distributing the burdens of proof', *Journal of Agricultural & Environmental Ethics*, 15(1): 103–122.

Wahlsten, D. (1999) 'Single-gene influences on brain and behavior', *Annual Review of Psychology*, 50: 599–624.

Warhurst, M. (2000) 'Crisis in chemicals: the threat posed by the biomedical revolution to the profits, liabilities and regulation of industries making and using chemicals', England, Wales and N. Ireland: Friends of the Earth, http://www.foe.co.uk/

pubsinfo/infoteam/pressrel/2000/20000605085125.html (accessed 30 October 2004).

Weatherall, D. (1999) 'From genotype to phenotype: genetics and medical practice in the new millennium', *Philosophical Transactions of the Royal Society: Biological Sciences*, 354: 1995–2010.

Wunder, M. (1999) 'Biomedicine and bioethics – the human being as optimisation project', http://bidok.uibk.ac.at/library/wunder-bio-e.html (accessed 10 Jan 2005).

Wunder, M. (2000) 'Medicine and conscience: the debate on medical ethics and research in Germany 50 years after Nuremberg', *Perspectives in Biology and Medicine*, 43: 373–381 (accessed 30 October 2004).

Chapter 11

Emerging forms of governance in genomics and post-genomics

Structures, trends, perspectives

Herbert Gottweis

Introduction

On 26 June 2000, at a White House ceremony, President Clinton appeared together with the director of the National Human Genome Project, Francis Collins, and the president of Celera Genomics, Craig Venter, to announce that the two groups had succeeded in almost completely decoding the human genome. President Clinton said that humanity had discovered nothing less than the language of God. Nobel prize winner James Watson predicted that this research would revolutionize society as much as Gutenberg´s printing press (*Financial Times*, 27 June 2000; *Herald Tribune*, 27 June 2000).

The HGP lies at the heart of the new scientific-technological field of genomics,[1] which focuses on the characterization and sequencing of the genome, and the analysis of the relationship between gene activity and cell function. While not everybody will agree with President Clinton´s or James Watson´s strong metaphoric language, there seems to be little disagreement in science, medicine, industry, mass media and the general public that the current advances in genomics will have a significant impact on medical practice, agriculture, economy, society and culture (Kitcher 1996). However, a considerable divergence in opinions exists today about how exactly genomics will exert its impact on science and society, who will benefit from the 'genomic revolution' (Abelson 1998) and what role governments and other institutions and actors such as private industry or patient groups should play to structure and guide the impact of genomics on society. Thus, Robert Dahl's (1961) classical question of 'Who Governs?' needs to be asked anew. The answer to this question is not clear at all, and this constitutes the central policy challenge for genomic governance. Who drives with which impact and legitimacy the pace of development and innovation in the field of genomics and post-genomics?

Governance is about the ways and means in which the divergent preferences of citizens are translated into effective policy choices, about how the plurality of social interests are transformed into unitary action and the compliance of actors is achieved (Rhodes 1997; Kohler-Koch and Eising 1999). The concept of governance stresses that state actors have lost their pivotal place above society (Pierre 2000). Today the political arena is populated by a multitude of autonomous actors who create patterns of structured co-operation despite the absence of a central organizing authority. Increasingly, local and national patterns of governance blend into transnational and global forms of policy-making. At the same time, new forms of governance emerge that take on a variety of forms that coexist in one and the same field. Unidirectional forms of governance such as top-down governance or bottom-up governance coexist with multidirectional forms of governance, such as network governance. In the field of genomics, 'traditional' governments or governmental institutions with a focus on top-down governance continue to play a crucial role in the support and regulation of research and development. At the same time bottom-up patterns of governance seem to emerge, as articulated by the increasing importance of patient groups or, more general, mass publics and public opinion in the shaping of genomics-related policy-making. Simultaneously, markets that steer horizontal exchanges between sellers and buyers, producers and consumers constitute important structural elements in the governance of genomics. Multidirectional forms of genomics governance have also taken on shape: we observe in the genomics field patterns of network governance, such as interactions and negotiation patterns between governments, non-governmental organizations and business alliances (Rosenau 2002: 80–81). This proliferation of patterns of governance, the location of governance on different levels from local to global, and the disaggregation of rule systems raises the question of the effectiveness, but also democratic quality of the emerging forms of governance in the field of genomics. Will tensions, conflicts and lack of co-ordination lead to crisis in the field of genomic governance?

In the following analysis I will reconstruct the emerging structures, patterns and levels of governance in the field of genomics, the rise of genomics from a scientific dream to a large-scale socio-technical project, the different ways genomic research has been supported and regulated by governmental agencies in a number of Western and non-Western countries, Further, I will discuss the rise of the genomics industry as a powerful force in the genomics governance network, the process by which genomics became a much admired, but also highly controversial public topic, and which future challenges can be expected in the governance of genomics.

From genomics to post-genomics

Genomics as a field of research embraces both the Human Genome Project (the world-wide programme to document the entire DNA sequence of the human genome) and the study of the relationship between genes and cell function in both health and disease (sometimes also called functional genomics). From a medical and pharmaceutical view, the importance of the HGP is based on the hope that it will provide the foundation for a comprehensive understanding of the relationship between genes and disease on two levels. First, the HGP will offer a new perspective on the relationship between genotype and disease. Based on data of the HGP, it will become possible to identify the genotypes which predispose individuals to a particular disease. Similarly, it might become possible to understand individual responses to therapies and thus to tailor treatments according to genetic profiles of patients. The field of pharmacogenomics focuses on the application of genomic technology to the discovery and development of drugs (Rothstein and Epps 2001: 228). Second, it is argued that the HGP will yield a new understanding of gene expression, of the specific genes which are active within a particular cell. Based on whole-genome information, functional genomics attempts to identify the patterns of gene expression which typify normal and diseased tissues. This, it is hoped, will help to find molecular markers for diagnosing and monitoring disease progression and to locate potential targets for therapeutic intervention (Collins et al. 1998; Schafer and Hawkins 1998; *Scripps Magazine*, February 1998: 32–36). In this respect, functional genomics can also be seen as representing the beginning of a 'post-genomic' era which moves on from the sequencing of genes to assigning some element of function to each of the genes in an organism.

Furthermore, the 'post-genomic' era seems to be characterized by a broad effort to move beyond strictly genetic determinism, to acknowledge the problematic genomic complexity, and to focus on expressed genes (proteins). In this perspective, genes do play a restricted role within living organisms; they do not actively direct metabolic processes or the activities of cells. Rather, according to the 'post-genomic' perspective the central players in the drama of molecular biology are in fact proteins. Thus, in the currently emerging (post-genomic) field of structural genomics, for example, interest focuses on the parts of the gene that are transcribed into messenger RNA, and so encode proteins. The idea behind what in the mean time is called the 'structural genomics initiative' is to discover and analyse the three-dimensional structures of protein, RNA and other biological macromolecules representing the entire range of structural diversity found in nature. Another new field, proteomics, constitutes an effort to identify all the proteins expressed in an organisms. Proteomics is based on the assumption that a cell′s full profile of proteins is not explicitly encoded by the genes and thus cannot be deciphered by analysis at the genetic level alone. To understand disease at the molecular level, it is necessary to look at the proteins directly (Parekh 1999; Abbott 2000). Thus, proteomics complements other functional genomics approaches and it is expected that the integration of these various data sets through bioinformatics will yield a comprehensive database of gene function (Tyers and Mann 2003: 193).

Ultimately, the strategic goals of genomics and post-genomics are far-reaching. As two researchers at the Howard Hughes Medical Institute have put it:

> Although the current research is focused on assigning function to genes and proteins, the long-term goal is just as it is for the child and the black box – that is, to be able to understand sufficiently well how the pieces work together and that you could, in principle, put them back together and get a functional organism.
>
> (Vukmirovic and Tilghman 2000: 822)

Central topics in the governance of genomics

Genomics and post-genomics represent a significant challenge for policy-making. Difficulties begin with the fact that it is not easy for policy-makers to figure out what exactly constitutes the challenge of genomics and post-genomics. Since the early 1980s the field has been moving rapidly ahead and every few months new initiatives and subdisciplines are presented, breakthroughs go hand in hand with setbacks, fantastic promises and enthusiastic forecasts do not only create optimism, but more than often are met with scepticism, in particular by the general public. Against this background of complexity, we can identify three interrelated areas of challenge in the governance of genomics: the promotion of genomics research and industry, the cultural and social dimensions of genomics, and risks and uncertainties associated with genomics.

Governing genomics I: issues of research and industrial development

The HGP emerged in the United States out of a number of unrelated sources in the mid-1980s. Initially the cost of the project was estimated to be around US$3 billion, a sum to be spread out over ten or twenty years, the expected duration of the project. From the outset it was clear that the HGP would initiate a new style of biology with its reliance on systematic technology development and centralized, goal-directed gene-mapping efforts. In 1990, after NIH and the Department of Energy had published their five-year mapping and sequencing plan for 1990–1995 and the National Center for Human Genome research had been established, criticism within the research community peaked. The main points of critique were that the HGP did not arise from a broad consensus among scientists but stemmed from more local, political interests; that the goals of the HGP were questionably focused on 'brute force sequencing' without specifically targeting diseases; and that the project would be divisive to the biomedical research community with its 'big science' versus 'little science' implications (Fortune 1993: 372–374; Cook-Deegan 1994).

With yearly allocations from Congress steadily rising from $59.5 million in 1990 to $218 million in 1998 and sequencing costs plummeting, the HGP continued to proceed within the forecasted expenses and received funding from eighteen other countries. In 1998 Celera Genomics announced that it intended to sequence the entire human genome by 2001 and patent many genes, a move which caused the HGP to speed up its own efforts (Coghlan and Boyce 2000). Though Celera's initiative was widely seen as bold and spectacular, it was also highly symbolic for the emergence of a world-wide operating genomics industry which attempted to integrate basic science with novel strategies to create new markets for new kinds of medical products. Following the example of the United States, we see today in many countries governmental or private initiatives in the context of human genome sequencing. For example, Britain's Wellcome Trust has been funding a programme at the Sanger Center that planned complete sequencing of one-third of the human genome. In Germany, the German Human Genome Project was launched with limited funds in 1996, with a 50% increase in funds to about $30 million in 2000. In 1999, France presented GenHomme, a five-year genomics programme to promote the creation of genomics start-ups and develop genomics technology platforms with the goal to develop new drugs, diagnostics and therapies. The central aim of the French project is to accelerate technology transfer and innovation from human genome data (Coghlan and Boyce 2000). During the late 1990s East Asia emerged as a new regional force in human genome research. For example, in 1998 China launched several major initiatives in human genomics with budgets totalling over $30 million (Triendl 2000). However, overall it must be said that developing countries lack the political will and the scientific and economic capacity to participate effectively in the Human Genome Project and its various spin-offs.

The mainly Western governmental and private efforts in genomics were to a considerable respect responsible for the gradual rise of a broadly based genomics industry with a significant number of new start-up companies involved in a variety of activities. While the 1990s saw the growth of companies in the area of sequencing, more recently companies focus on gene function, its variability (i.e. single nucleotide polymorphisms or SNPs) and pharmacogenomics with the idea to eventually develop successfully new drugs (Asia Pacific Biotech 2003: 707). Since the early 1990s, a number of major companies developed in the field of genomics industry of which the most important are Millennium Pharmaceuticals, Human Genome Sciences, Celera Genomics, Incyte Genomics and Affymetrix.

Emblematic in this context is the company Celera, the leading private player in the creation of a 'working draft' of the human genome. Recently Celera also announced a major effort in proteomics. Celera's move mirrored a march of genomics companies into proteomics and the dawn of post-genomics. Today virtually every major pharmaceutical company has a proteomics effort under way. In the current proteomics rush, most companies are taking more or less the same brute force approach to determine which proteins are present in various tissues (Science 2000). One important research product in genomics research and industry is SNPs: 99.9% of the human DNA sequence is shared by all humans, but the final 0.1% differs from one individual to the other. The sites where these differences occur are known as single nucleotide polymorphisms. Each individual has a unique combination of polymorphisms. In April 1999 a consortium of pharmaceutical companies, genome research institutions and the Wellcome Trust announced that they would work together to produce a public database of SNPs. In addition to these research efforts, a number of biopharmaceutical companies active in genomics are searching for genes involved in common diseases, both for developing new drug targets and for laying the foundation for pharmacogenomics (Oxagen, UK; DeCODE, Iceland) (Schafer and Hawkins 1998; Wellcome Trust News 1999).

In general, just like in the rest of biotech development, more and more technological and scientific advancements are the result of collaboration on a global scale. While the sequencing of the human genome was completed by Celera Genomics and the US-government-sponsored Human Genome Project, and the core of the work was performed in the United States and in the United Kingdom, the international human genome sequencing consortium included scientists at sixteen institutions across France, Germany, Japan and China (Ernst and Young 2001). A similar picture develops in the biggest follow-up project to the sequencing effort of the 1990s: the HapMap project. Launched in 2002, it will chart genetic variation within the human genome. The central idea of the HapMap project is to create a human haplotype map. In the cell divisions, pairs of chromosomes line up and exchange portions of genetic material. This process is not entirely random because the breaking, exchange and resealing tend to occur at particular points. As a result, blocks of sequence have been inherited down the generations. These blocks are known as haplotypes. The HapMap then would allow geneticists to scan the entire genome rapidly for disease genes by analysing some 300,000 SNPs (as compared to some 10 million common SNPs scattered throughout the human genome). To create the HapMap, DNA will be taken from blood samples from Nigeria, Japan, China and the United States. Public funding for the effort will be provided by the Japanese Ministry of Education, Culture, Sports, Science and Technology; Genome Canada in Ottawa and Genome Quebec in Montreal; the Chinese Academy of Sciences, the Chinese Ministry of Science and Technology, and the Natural Science Foundation of China; and the US National Institutes of Health (NIH). The SNP Consortium (TSC) in Deerfield, IL, will co-ordinate private funding, while the Wellcome Trust in London will provide charitable funding for the United Kingdom portion of the project (Dennis 2003: 758).

While stock prices of genomics companies are rising across the board, the prospects of these companies will alter rapidly over the next few years as publicly funded projects in genomic sequencing and SNP mapping reduce the value of raw data. Genomics companies will have to persuade pharmaceutical firms that it is their approach, rather than any other, that will make drug discovery and development faster or cheaper or more effective (or all three) (James 2000).

The picture of the unfolding structure for governance in genomic and post-genomic research and industry is the following: in the United States, in Europe and in East Asia governments are strong players in genomics. There is a certain tendency for national initiatives in the field, but also for close international collaboration. The strong position of private companies is a further key feature in shaping the newly emerging governance structure, companies which either compete with government strategies (HGP) or collaborate (SNP initiative). The new situation also influences the choice of subjects. As predicted by critics in the early 1990s, the era when scientists decided about the direction of their research seems to be history. Scientists are now obliged to respond to calls for tenders issued by governments, the European Union and large companies following economic and business-strategic criteria. Not only is the boundary between business and academia blurred by definition, but also there is a new line of demarcation appearing separating government and academic scientists in large centres able to respond to calls for tenders, and others, who increasingly are not part of this new game in biology. The result is not only the shaping of a new industrial or governmental complex, but also a fundamental transformation of biology far beyond the initial Human Genome Project initiative, as indicated by post-genomics projects such as proteomics and structural genomics. The combined process of concentration and top-down definition of research goals seems to continue in the 'follow-up' projects to the human genome initiative. While the HGP was defined by the scalable task of DNA sequencing and the attending technologies such as polymerase chain reaction and automated sequencing, proteomics has to deal with problems such as limited and variable sample material, sample degradation, vast dynamic range and almost boundless tissue, developmental and temporal specificity. 'While proteomics is by definition expected to yield direct biological insights, all of these difficulties render any comprehensive proteomics projects an inherently intimidating and often humbling exercise' (Tyers and Mann 2003: 193).

Obviously, these developments raise a number of important ethical and social governance issues, which will be discussed in the following sections. But they also raise a number of critical questions concerning the forces that direct contemporary development in the life sciences, and the consequences of this development. On the one hand, there seems to be a vast, global public/private effort under its way to revolutionize the current practice of biomedical research and health care. However, it should not be ignored that fundamental critique concerning the described transformation of biology continues. Many scientists are deeply concerned about the current transformation of modern biology from being driven by the interest of individual scientists to a 'Big Science' discipline. In addition, eminent scientists such as Richard C. Strohman have deeply questioned the continuing genetic determinism underlying large-scale projects such as the HGP and its follow-up projects and their implicit rejection of more holistic considerations of ways to go from the genome to complex biological function. According to Strohman (1997) it will be necessary to move away from a focus on genetic and protein agents per se toward their interaction with networks and emergent features of networks such as distributed control and openness to local and environmental signals. Critics have also pointed to the failure of gene therapy as a proof for the limited value of genomic research. Furthermore, some voices in the discussion emphasized the multifactorial character of diseases and thus, the limited chances of tailor-made pharmaceuticals (*Scripps Magazine*, June 2000: 18). Taking into account the recent history of new biotechnology, its profound and continuing failure to deliver on the level of products, and its possible epistemological limitations, such criticism should not be taken lightly by research support agencies, in particular with respect to the direction of their funding policies.

Thus, genomic governance in the research and industry domain seems to be characterized by a dynamics operating on a global level with governments having become co-operation or conflict partners of private companies and consortia of scientists networking. The resulting new genomic governance networks have created a new dynamics of scientific-technological change that seems to question local and national democratic negotiation of scientific development and also challenge the effectiveness of political scrutiny by nationally elected representative institutions.

Governing genomics II: cultural issues

The essence of governance is to reach social compromise and binding decisions. Hence, democratic regimes of governance in the field of genomics comprise not only policy-makers, scientists and entrepreneurs, but also patients, consumers, the general public and the mass media. At first glance medical biotechnology seems to enjoy solid support by the general public. Survey research shows quite clearly that – despite increasing opposition to agricultural biotechnology – there is strong public support for the various medical applications of genomics from genetic testing to pharmaceuticals (Gaskell et al. 2000; Priest 2000). However, in the early 1990s the future also looked bright for agricultural biotechnology. In a similar way, Frankendrugs and Frankencells could appear quickly on the horizon of public concern.

There are a number of well-defined reasons why opposition against genomics could become stronger. The case of genetic discrimination is a good example in this context, a topic I will discuss below. But it needs to be emphasized that at this point in time we also seem to be witnessing a more basic development in the public perception of genomics. This development has more to do with general beliefs and world-views than with specific concerns about implications of genomics. On the most fundamental level, genomics and post-genomics seem to offer an image of humankind and with it a new techno-scientific imagery, which represents humans as determined by their genes and, at the same time, portrays human genes as objects of technological manipulation and transformation. Even if only a few maverick scientists speculate about the point when genomics scientists will be able to build 'organisms from the scratch', it is precisely such speculations which are gladly taken up by the mass media and disseminated to a broad public. Craig Venter's intensively discussed experiments to determine the number of genes needed for *Mycoplasma genitalium* to survive found its way directly into the headline of the *Scotsman* in the following form: 'Frankencell Gene Team Accused of Playing God' (quoted in Harris 2000: 128). While most scientists in genomics will reject the idea that they have any intention to 'play God', they increasingly cannot escape their new image as being in the business of 'human engineering', which increasingly seems to dominate public fantasies and belief systems. The identification of DNA with 'the human person' has made 'life' problematic because this definition escapes the currently available self-understandings provided by both the classical world and the Christian tradition (Rabinow 1999). As a result, a 'cultural vacuum' seems to exist, which gives room for many, sometimes wild, speculations about the meaning and goals of contemporary genomics. It is against this background that I consider growing and unspecific opposition against genomics as a possible scenario. In the future this opposition could be strengthened by a public perception of genomics as being associated with other controversial fields, such as therapeutic cloning and human, embryonic stem cell research.

Governing genomics III: regulatory issues

As I mentioned, at this point in time neither in the United States nor in Europe nor elsewhere can we witness strong public opposition against genomics. In the case of opposition against genomics growing, I consider it to be unlikely that much of this opposition will be directed against genomics research and industry per se. People might have generalized anxieties about genomic medicine, but for these anxieties to become political they must be translated into a well-structured topic of controversy. Most likely, for most citizens and groups 'genomics as such' will be too abstract to lend itself to focused political mobilization. In the period since the late 1970s, genetic engineering debates have supported this interpretation. During the second half of the 1970s opposition against genetic engineering did not focus on research policies, but on regulatory topics. A similar picture can be observed in the case of agricultural biotechnology (Gottweis 1998). Hence, based on currently observable tendencies, I expect criticism of genomics to be located in a number of different arenas of governance of which the most important are the regulation of patenting, of genetic testing, gene therapy, genomic medicine and the corresponding topics of individual privacy protection, genetic information, genetic discrimination, protection of research volunteers, and access to genomic services (Sharp et al. 2004: 4).

Patenting

Since the early 1990s patenting has become a central topic in the governance of genomics. Many voices in industry and science argue that people working in the field of genetics make discoveries and the granting of patents will encourage them to make their findings public. The counterargument is that DNA should not be patentable at all because nobody invented it. This argument has not impressed the US Supreme Court, which ruled in 1990 in its Diamond v. Chakrabarty decision, that genetically modified bacteria were patentable. Today the US Patent and Trademark Office (PTO) holds that even 'natural' DNA as a chemical compound, once isolated and purified, is patentable. Thus, the US PTO and the European Patent Office (EPO) have treated isolated and purified nucleoide sequences as if they were the same as synthetic chemicals (Andrews 2002: 803). To date the PTO has issued more than 2000 patents on full-length genes and many more applications have come in. Human Genome Sciences has filed applications encompassing 7500 full-length genes. The French company Genset SA has generated over 90,000 sequences of 5-prime untranslated region sequence tags of human full-length cDNA clones and patent applications will be filed.[2]

Within the research community the main concern is that the patenting of genes will not only reward research efforts, but also hinder the exploitation of newly discovered functions for DNA sequences, prevent testing services, create obstacles for product developments, and, in general stifle research and development. The Human Genome Organization (HUGO), for example, states that it welcomes initiatives such as those by the SNPs consortium to map all SNPs and to put them in the public domain. Furthermore, HUGO underscores that any DNA molecule and sequence without unambiguous indication and disclosure of its function should not be patentable (HUGO 2000). This critique within the genomics community is mirrored by the general public, where a general feeling of uneasiness seems to exist concerning the patenting of genes. Part of this critical attitude is caused by a generalized fear that patents will enable companies to own people's genes (Gold 2000). When companies began to insist on their patent rights in the context of genetic testing, soon fierce controversy erupted. For example, Athena Neurosciences holds a patent on a gene that is associated with Alzheimer diseases and does not allow any laboratory except its own to screen for the mutation of this gene. In 2001 Myriad Genetics (USA) was granted a European patent related to the *BRCA1* breast cancer associated gene and, consequentially, had disputed the right of French doctors to test for *BRCA1* mutations. It required that all test samples be sent to its laboratory. This has led to challenges in the courts (Andrews 2002: 804). In both cases outraged publics and researchers questioned the companies' demands as conflicting with the basic rules of patient care. In Europe the Institut Curie in France challenged Myriad Genetics' European patent and were joined by the governments of Belgium and the Netherlands (Andrews 2002: 806). In the United States, a bill submitted before Congress in 2002 would exempt from patent infringement medical practitioners who perform genetic diagnostic tests based on patented gene sequences (Chahine 2002). In 2002 the British Nuffield Council on Bioethics recommended that patents on genetic sequences should be the exception rather than the rule, a position that has also found sympathy in other countries such as Canada and France (*Nature* 2003). Overall the patenting issue in genomics is far from settled and will constitute a field of controversy for many years to come. With massive projects in the field of proteomics under way, the question of patents on proteins and biological molecules seems to open up a new field of claims and controversy. Again, such claims might create considerable obstacles for research, testing and therapy (Cyranoski 2003). While the most important policy actors in the field of patenting, the US PTO and the EPO have advocated a positive approach towards gene patents, it seems that a number of national governments, together with scientists, medical doctors and concerned publics have begun to challenge the strategy of the major national patent offices.

Genetic testing, genetic information and beyond

The great hype around genomics is based not simply on the impression that genomic research will enable humanity to develop a completely new understanding of the 'blueprint of life'. As mentioned above, much of the industrial, scientific and political interest in genomics has to do with the expectation that the insights of genomics can be used not only to better understand health and disease, but also to develop novel medical strategies to cure and/or to prevent disease. The standard economic interpretation of genomics goes like this: those companies who are able to use genomic knowledge for therapeutic or preventive purposes will – protected by corresponding patent legislation – be in a position to open up new medical markets with substantial growth potentials (Enriquez 1998).

The main areas for the application of genomics can be found in the following areas: first, based on genetic testing, novel information about predisposition to diseases can be gathered. Obviously, the data from the HGP are critical for developing these new tests. Once this novel patient information is available, predisposition to particular diseases can be determined and potential responses to therapies be predicted. Second, the new information based on genetic testing will open up a new field of tailored treatment (pharmacogenomics). Third, based on data from the HGP, therapeutic interventions on the genetic level will systematically improve, and in particular open up new possibilities for gene therapy (Parekh 1999).

Currently, gene therapy is still in its infancy and suffers from a history of failures and accidents. Apparently, the complexities of medical intervention on the level of human genes have been underestimated and most clinical trials in this field are in their first stages (Abbott 2001). The potential ethical-social implications of gene therapy, in particular of germline therapy, are enormous, and broadly discussed in the United States and in Europe. However, at this point in time these debates are largely theoretical due to gene therapy's sobering lack of success to actually cure diseases (National Reference Center for Bioethics Literature 2000).

In contrast, genetic testing has clearly emerged as both a new medical sub-industry with a huge market potential and a broadly applied medical technology based on research in genomics. More than 400 genetic tests are currently available. Genetic testing includes predicting the risk of disease, identifying carriers and establishing prenatal diagnosis and prognosis. For several years, the United States has been flooded with tests which screen for the genetic mutations predisposing patients for certain diseases. The spectrum of the targeted pathologies seems limitless ranging from tests for the predisposition of osteoporosis to breast cancer. The US company PPGx has began to market a test for alleles that confer slow drug metabolism directly to the public to give patients the possibility of directing their own treatment.[3]

The socio-political and ethical implications of this new medical culture of testing and information gathering are multifold. Concerns exist with respect to the problem of genetic discrimination, the gap between genetic information and prediction and available therapies, and the potential rise of a new form of eugenics based either on the pooling of information or abuse of data from prenatal screening. Fears about genetic discrimination in the workplace exist in the United States as much as in Europe. A US survey shows that 85% of US citizens believe that employers should be prohibited from obtaining information about an individual's genetic conditions, risks and predispositions. Workplace-related genetic tests seem to be more widespread in the United States than in Europe. According to a 1999 survey, 30% of the large and midsize companies in the United States sought some form of information about their employees and 7% used this information in awarding promotions and hiring. This process seems to accelerate as the costs of DNA testing go down. Since the 1990s more than a hundred federal and state legislative efforts to protect employees against genetic discrimination have been shelved by US legislators. However, in 2000 President Clinton signed an executive order forbidding the use of genetic testing in the hiring of federal employees (Martindale 2001). The legal situation is equally ambiguous in Europe. While in most countries there are a number of laws which in principle could be used to protect against genetic discrimination (United Kingdom, Germany), only a few countries have specific legislation focused on genetic testing (Switzerland, the Netherlands, France).

The public is furthermore strongly concerned that genetic information will be used by insurers to deny, limit or cancel health insurance. Survey research shows that 85% of Americans thought that health insurers should be barred from accessing genetic information. At this point in time the problem of health insurance discrimination seems to be more discussed in the United States, where private health insurance is the rule, as compared to Europe where most countries have public health insurance. In the United States the Health Insurance Portability and Accountability Act (HIPAA) 1996 was a first important step countering the possibility of health insurance discrimination based on genetic information. Further legislative steps to close HIPAA loopholes are in preparation (Martindale 2001).

Another field of concern is large-scale random population genotyping, which might allow companies to gain information about future morbidity and the structure and size of health care markets. In this context the most important questions are should such a stock of information be generated at all? And how could safeguards be developed to keep such sensitive information confidential and avoid abuse?

Finally, the ever-increasing number of prenatal tests, including preimplantation diagnosis (PID), raises a whole spectrum of questions. Concerns exist with respect of a possible increase of selective abortions based on genetic testing and the rise of a 'new form of eugenics'. While genetic testing has a long tradition in medicine, human genome research has led to the rapid detection of many more mutated genes that are involved in a number of human diseases and disorders. This could lead to a thorough redefinition of the boundary between health and disease and corresponding implications for genetic counselling. Furthermore, the coupling of the new (genomic) knowledge with rapid developments in reproductive technologies raises the spectrum of the modification of human germline cells, in particular in the context of in vitro fertilization and PID (Andrews 1999).

So far the concerns of patients and consumer groups about applications and practices of genomics from patenting to testing and information gathering have been insufficiently addressed by policy-makers in the United States and Europe. Today virtually everybody involved in the science, business and politics of genomics readily agrees that genomics raises many ethical, moral and social issues. United States funding of research about the social and ethical sides of genomics by ELSI has created a wealth of data and ideas about how to deal with the new challenges in genomics. However, these insights and critical evaluations have not yet been followed adequately by corresponding regulatory measures or institutional designs. In the United States, for example, no regulation exists to evaluate genetic tests. Nearly all genetic tests bypass the Food and Drug Administration (FDA) because most of these new tests are categorized as services which the FDA does not regulate (*Nature Medicine* 2003). The DNA patenting race continues and current legislation and court decisions in Europe and in the United States have contributed to its further acceleration. The genetic testing industry is booming and in most Western countries policy-makers have been reluctant to impose regulatory measures dealing with workplace testing. As a result, genomic technologies are in the process of accumulating a vast amount of genetic information which is only insufficiently protected from abuse. However, there are some reassuring signs. After seven years' negotiation, the US Senate has unanimously passed the Genetic Information Nondiscrimination Act 2003, which is to prohibit the use of genetic information by insurers or employers. In Europe, an expert group of the European Commission released a report on genetic testing in which a comprehensive framework for the regulation of genetic testing in Europe was outlined (European Commission 2004). However, much regulatory action still needs to be taken in the field of genomics.

A good example is the understudied field of pharmacogenomics regulation. Assuming that the vision of 'personalized medicine' will eventually materialize, a complex set of regulatory challenges will have to be addressed. As the number of pharmacogenomic drugs on the market increase, physicians might become responsible for prescribing the appropriate class of drug, but pharmacists would be determining the drug sub-type and dosage for maximum efficacy. A new system of patient health management would evolve, for example with important implications for liability. These issues have moved only gradually into the focus of regulatory interest (Rothstein and Epps 2001).

Conclusion

In this chapter I have argued that the science of genomics is in the process of introducing a number of fundamental transformations in the practices of modern biology and medicine, in pharmaceutical industry, in society and culture. In democracy, ideally, such a process is negotiated between the various affected and involved groups in order to create legitimacy, understanding and trust for the evolving structures of governance.

When in the mid-1980s the idea of a Human Genome Project began to take shape, there was widespread criticism within the scientific community about the possibly negative impacts of the HGP on the direction and style of modern biomedical research. The main concerns of the critics were genomics' narrow focus on genetic causality and its lack of interest in organismic complexity. In the mean time, scientific progress in modern biology and, closely related, modern biomedicine, is increasingly defined by large-scale projects such as the HGP or, recently, various initiatives in proteomics. These big science projects are quickly changing the modes and practices of scientific inquiry in modern biology. The new dynamics of developments in genomics and post-genomics is to a large extent made possible by the operation of a powerful coalition of government, industry and big science interests. Small genomics start-up companies compete with public research bodies in order to win financial offers from pharmaceutical companies. Research goals in basic science are not selected any more on the base of purely academic considerations, but guided by considerations of economic benefit. Finally, the key actors in this game have played an important role to considerably extend the role of patent rights in the field of modern biology and biomedicine. The governance of genomics seems to be shaped by a new culture which redefines the classical roles of government, industry and science in scientific-technological development. The state is only one actor next to many others in the shaping of biomedical futures. Finally, the governance of genomics clearly transcends the local and national sphere and operates economically, socially and politically on a global level.

The transformative powers of genomics and post-genomics have created a significant number of interrelated policy challenges in most Western countries. So far, these new topics of governance are only gradually being taken up in the already operating or emerging institutional structures of politics. There exists a gap between policy challenges and institutional responses. The existing institutions either fail to deal adequately with the new regulatory issues raised by genomics – or they still need to be created to face up to the new policy issues. In policy-making, such constellations of 'institutional void' often lead to policy conflicts, crises and social turbulences. Hence, it should not come as a surprise if stronger criticism of the political-regulatory handling of genomics and, on a more general level, of the science of genomics should materialize in the near future. A scenario of medical biotechnology repeating the fate of agricultural biotechnology is conceivable.

Growth of social, cultural and political opposition against genomics and post-genomics and, in particular, genomic medicine could take different forms. The first scenario is a relatively 'calm' one. No doubt, many patients and patient groups will be happy to profit from the various therapies and technologies offered by genomics and post-genomics whatever their ethical or moral consequences might be. This large segment of the population will most likely correspond with those who subscribe fully to the ideas and the practices of modern medicine. However, already now a growing number of patients have turned away from contemporary, modern medicine and are seeking alternatives. This is clearly indicated by the booming sector of alternative medicine. A growing number of people feel disaffected by the strictures of scientific medicine and embrace alternative therapies which eschew the use of high technology and laboratory data collection. This is as much an expression of disillusionment as of a cultural shift (Goldstein 1999). Obviously, those who already prefer homeopathic pills over antibiotics will not be easily persuaded of the benefits of genetic breast cancer testing. They will become convinced of the benefits of genomics neither by 'more public information' (one of the great myths of biotechnology policy), nor by new 'wonderdrugs', nor by new regulatory structures allowing for more public participation in the field of genomics. The 'alternative segment' of the population might 'vote with its feet' against genomics by allocating individual health budgets to the sector of alternative medicine. This group might also be inclined to give their votes at political elections to those parties and candidates which promise a reorientation in medical research spending.

The second scenario for opposition against genomics and post-genomics could follow a more familiar road. In this scenario genomic medicine would become more explicitly a topic for dissent. Certain developments such as genetic discrimination at the workplace might be targeted by critics and become a topic for political demands. As a result pressure might rise to introduce regulatory measures and improve public participation in the governance of genomics, for example by giving labour unions more influence in genetic testing decisions at the company level. Likewise, health insurance discrimination could lead to demands for strict legislation protecting employees from abuse of genetic information.

Finally, a situation might develop where a scandal or an accident related to genomics, for example widespread genetic data abuse or accidents related to products of pharmacogenetics might lead to a more fundamental rejection or fundamental questioning of genomics and post-genomics even by those, who, in principle, are sympathetic to the idea of modern medicine. The impact of the BSE disaster on agricultural policy in Germany, Austria and other European countries might offer a good comparison in this context.

Obviously, these three scenarios of rising opposition to medical genomics do not exclude each other. Currently we already see in a number of countries traces of the first two scenarios. But opposition against genomic medicine has not yet reached the threshold of fully developed political controversy. For this to happen elements of the three opposition scenarios need to coincide. For example, growing generalized concerns about genomics lead to more specific demands for legislative action. In such a situation, some sort of genomics-related scandal, for example in the context of drug-development, erupts which seems to confirm people's worst anxieties and concerns about genomics. It does not need much fantasy to imagine how in the wake of this development, public opinion begins to turn against genomic medicine, just as it happened in the field of agricultural biotechnology.

Who, then, governs the field of genomics and post-genomics? Which forces determine the pace of scientific and technological development and how are these processes related to political steering and negotiation? One result from my analysis is that national governments and policy-making clearly have lost importance and influence in the governance of genomics and post-genomics in the context of the emerging, multidirectional patterns of network governance. But this certainly does not imply that states or governments do not or could not actively engage in shaping scientific-technological development in the life sciences. In fact, such policies on the national level, in particular in the regulatory field, might be crucial for the future of genomics. The emerging regimes of patenting in the field of genomics are a good case in point where national actors from science, governments or parliaments have actively taken part in court challenges to gene patents. Governments continue to be crucial actors in supporting research and development in genomics research, as most recently evidenced by the HapMap project. Also, in most countries national regulatory regimes dealing with the genetic testing and information complex still urgently need to be created, in particular with respect to post-genomic projects, such as pharmacogenomics. There is little evidence that the necessary regulatory structures in many sub-fields of genomic governance will soon be created on a transnational level. But the development of such regulatory regimes will be crucial to create public support and acceptance of the new genomic technologies.

Ideally, the designs of these regulatory regimes would be discursive, open for horizontal interaction between the key actors involved in regulation, and also link science with politics and the public. Such structures could play a critical role to establish trust in the governance of genomics. Today, trust, be it in politics or in science, cannot be any longer assumed (Putnam 1993). Policy-making activities such as shaping regulations for genetic testing are not simply about finding solutions for problems, they are as much about finding formats that generate trust among mutually interdependent actors. Furthermore, novel ways should be devised to initiate a broadly based public dialogue and negotiation about the culture and practices of genomics. This dialogue should not be misconstrued as a mechanism to educate or inform the public (Bensaude-Vincent 2001). In the past most efforts in this direction in biotechnology have failed miserably. Rather, such a public dialogue and negotiation must be an honest and open effort to deal with the cultural vacuum created by the socio-technical project of genomics and post-genomics.

While in the emerging regimes of governance in genomics and post-genomics national policy-making still has an important role to play, it needs to be seen that any actor in genomic and post-genomic governance operates within a global system. The major research and development support policy initiatives in the genomics and post-genomics field give evidence that national policy-makers have fully acknowledged the interdependent and global character of contemporary research in genomics. That being the case, in the future national policy-makers and governments will also have to put emphasis on the supra- and transnational co-ordination of their regulatory efforts in order to establish an efficient counterweight and balance to the activities and interventions of industry, science and non-governmental organizations in shaping genomics and post-genomics governance today.

Notes

1 In this chapter I will focus on human genomics and not discuss genomic research in plant and animal sciences.
2 *Wall Street Journal* (2000) 'Own the genome? Genes are patentable. Less clear is what the finder needs to know', *Wall Street Journal*, 17 March; Meek, J. (2000) 'The race to buy life', *Guardian*, 15 November.
3 See *Biofuture*, February 2000: 66; *BioCentury, The Bernstein Report on BioBusiness*, 13 November 2000: 10.

References

Abbott, A. (2000) 'Structures by numbers', *Nature,* 408: 130–132.
Abbott, A. (2001) 'Genetic medicine gets real', *Nature*, 411: 410–412.
Abelson, P.H. (1998) 'A third technological revolution', *Science,* 27 March: 2019.
Andrews, L.B. (1999) *The Clone Age: Adventures in the New World of Reproductive Technology*. New York: Henry Holt.
Andrews, L.B. (2002) 'Genes and patent policy: rethinking intellectual property rights', *Nature Reviews Genetics*, 3: 803–808.
Asia Pacific Biotech (2003) 'Market overview', *Asia Pacific Biotech*, 7: 705–707.
Bensaude-Vincent, B. (2001) 'A genealogy of the increasing gap between science and the public', *Public Understanding of Science*, 10: 99–113.
Chahine, K. (2002) 'Industry opposes genomic legislation', *Nature Biotechnology*, 20: 419.
Coghlan, A. and Boyce, N. (2000) 'The end of the beginning: the first draft of the human genome signals a new area for humanity', *New Scientist*, 1 July: 4–5.
Collins, F.S., Patrinos, A., Jordan, E., Chakravarti, A., Gesteland, R. and Walters, L.R. (1998) 'New goals for the U.S. Human Genome Project: 1998–2003', *Science*, 282: 682–687.
Cook-Deegan, R. (1994) *The Gene Wars: Science, Politics, and the Human Genome*. London: Norton.
Cyranoski, D. (2003) 'This protein belongs to . . .', *Nature*, 426: 10–11.
Dahl, R.D. (1961) *Who Governs?* New Haven, CT: Yale University Press.
Dennis, C. (2003) 'The rough guide to the genome', *Nature*, 425: 758–759.
Enriquez, J. (1998) 'Genomics and the world's economy', *Science*, 281: 925–926.

Ernst and Young (2001) *Focus on Fundamentals: The Biotechnology Report*, 88. London.

European Commission (2004) *25 Recommendations on the Ethical, Legal, and Social Implications of Genetic Testing*. Brussels: EC.

European Community, Official Journal (1998) Directive 98/44/EC of the European Parliament and the Council of 6 July 1998 on the Legal Protection of Biotechnology Inventions, 30 July: 13–21.

Fortune, M. (1993) 'Mapping and making genes and histories: the Genomics Project in the United States 1980–1990', PhD Dissertation, Harvard University, Cambridge, MA.

Gaskell, G., Bauer, M.W., Allum, N. and Durant, J. (2000) 'Biotechnology and the European public', *Nature Biotechnology*, 18: 935–938.

Gold, R.E. (2000) 'Moving the gene patent debate forward: a framework for achieving compromise between industry and civil society', *Science*, 18: 1319–1320.

Goldstein, M. (1999) *Alternative Health Care: Medicine, Miracle, or Mirage?* Philadelphia, PA: Temple University Press.

Gottweis, H. (1998) *Governing Molecules: The Discursive Politics of Genetic Engineering in Europe and in the United States*. Cambridge, MA: MIT Press.

Harris, R. (2000) 'Frankencells and mirth', *Current Biology*, 10(4): 128.

HUGO (2000) Memo, London.

James, R. (2000) 'Differentiating genomics companies', *Nature Biotechnology*, 13: 153–155.

Kitcher, P. (1996) *The Lives to Come: The Genetic Revolution and Human Possibilities*. London: Penguin.

Kohler-Koch, B. and Eising, R. (eds) (1999) *The Transformation of Governance in the European Union*. London: Routledge.

Martindale, D. (2001) 'Pink slip in your genes', *Scientific American*, January: 13–14.

National Reference Center for Bioethics Literature (2000) *Human Gene Therapy*. Scope Note 24, February.

Nature (2000) 'German government takes a narrow view of gene patents', *Nature*, 406: 664.

Nature (2003) 'Gene patents and the public good', *Nature*, 423: 207.

Nature Medicine (2003) 'Getting a grip on genetic testing' (editorial), *Nature Medicine*, 9: 147.

Parekh, R. (1999) 'Proteomics and molecular medicine', *Nature Biotechnology*, 17: 267–268.

Pierre, J. (ed.) (2000) *Debating Governance: Authority, Steering, and Democracy*. Oxford: Oxford University Press.

Priest, S.H. (2000) 'US public opinion divided over biotechnology?', *Nature Biotechnology*, 18: 939–942.

Putnam, R. (1993) *Making Democracy Work: Civic Traditions in Modern Italy*. Princeton, NJ: Princeton University Press.

Rabinow, P. (1999) *French DNA: Trouble in Purgatory*. Chicago, IL: University of Chicago Press.

Rhodes, R.A.W. (1997) *Understanding Governance. Policy Networks, Governance, Reflexivity and Accountability*. Buckingham: Open University Press.

Rosenau, J.N. (2002) 'Governance in a new global order', in D. Held and A. McGrew (eds) *Governing Globalization: Power, Authority and Global Governance*. Cambridge: Polity Press.

Rothstein, M.A. and Epps, P.G. (2001) 'Ethical and legal implications of pharmacogenomics', *Nature Review Genetics*, 2 (March): 228–221.

Schafer, A.J. and Hawkins, J.R. (1998) 'DNA variations and the future of human genetics', *Nature Biotechnology*, 16: 33–38.

Science (2000) 287: 2136–2138.

Sharp, R.R., Yudell, M.A. and Wilson, S.H. (2004) 'Shaping science policy in the age of genomics', *Nature Reviews Genetics*, 5: 1–9.

Strohman, R.C. (1997) 'Profit margins and epistemology', *Nature Biotechnology*, 15: 1224–1225.

Triendl, R. (2000) 'Genomics forges ahead in East Asia', *Nature Biotechnology* 18: 278–279.

Tyers, M. and Mann, M. (2003) 'From genomics to proteomics', *Nature*, 422: 193–197.

Vukmirovic, O.G. and Tilghman, S.M. (2000) 'Exploring genome space', *Nature*, 405: 821–822.

Wellcome Trust News (1999) '"Q 3", the cutting edge. SNPs and their medical application', *Wellcome Trust News*, 14–15.

Index